MORE CHOCOLATE, NO CAVITIES

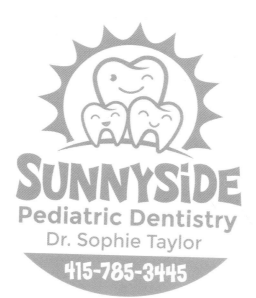

MORE CHOCOLATE, NO CAVITIES

How Diet Can Keep Your Kid Cavity-Free

Dr. Roger W. Lucas DDS

Pediatric Dentist, Bachelor of Science in Biochemistry

ISBN-13: 9781517705497
ISBN-10: 1517705495
Library of Congress Control Number: 2015916615
CreateSpace Independent Publishing Platform
North Charleston, South Carolina

Disclaimer: This book provides general information and does not create any patient-physician relationship and should not be used as a substitute for professional diagnosis and treatment. You should consult with your child's physician, dentist, registered dietician, and/or other health care provider with questions and/or making any major decisions regarding diet or other health issues. You should not disregard professional medical advice or delay seeking it because of what you might have read in this book. The information contained herein is provided "as is" and without warranty of any kind.

This book is dedicated to:
My wife,
Who has supported me over
12 years of marriage.

My daughters,
Who inspired me to start doing the research.

My patients' families,
Thanks for everything you have taught me and for
giving me the best job in the world.

Acknowledgements

Thanks first to my developmental editor, Barbara Mulvey Little (BarbaraMulveyLittle.com). Barbara did such excellent work in helping my science brain get things straight. Wendy Amara and Shanna Pearson (OneFocusTotalSuccess.com), Wendy in particular for saving my marriage (no big deal) and helping me finish this book. (Maybe I should put her first?) Dr. Philippe Hujoel (University of Washington School of Dentistry) for not being afraid of fat back in 2009 before it was cool. Tim Grahl (TimGrahl.com) for teaching me to be relentlessly helpful and commit to writing to help the world. Beth Jusino (BethJusino.com), my consulting editor. Thanks for giving me real-world feedback. Dr. John Gottman (gottman.com), thanks for spending one minute with me to answer a question after a lecture, and for helping me stay married for 12 years. John Medina (JohnMedina.com) for teaching to me to talk fast at a lecture at UPC, and for lectures on raising kids. Jonathan Catherman (jonathancatherman.com) for how to cook a steak, and being a great mentor in my youth. Dan Pink (DanPink.com) for teaching me that "sometimes you have to write to figure it out." Clifton Griffin and Janine Coleman (https://cgd.io/) for making my website and for graphic design. Thanks to Evergreen Study Club for giving me helpful feedback on my topic. Thanks to Dr. Travis Nelson for the original snack guide inspiration.

Thanks especially to the beta readers. Your feedback (good and bad) was invaluable: Quinn Manning, Marcella Nichols, Alicia Wong, Mai Le, Penelope Wright, Jeanine Layes, Avanti Bergquist, Brandon Swervo, Mike Grodin, Ryan Chiang, Cathie Coffin, Marena Newhouse, Wanda Claro.

Table of Contents

Ask the right questions.

In dental school, we asked the question, how do we reduce cavities?

Then my wife and I had children of our own. I saw some of my doctor and dentist friends whose children had unexplained cavities despite the parents' best efforts. I wanted to ask a new question: How do I keep my kids completely cavity-free, even if both her mom and I had several cavities growing up? Someone please tell me exactly what to do. I don't want my kids to have fifty percent less cavities. I want them to have zero cavities. Fluoride reduces cavities. Brushing reduces cavities. Flossing reduces cavities. But it wasn't always enough.

My wife, not being a dentist but more of a realist, had a different type of question: How do I keep my kids cavity-free without insane amounts of effort?

I want to make my wife happy.

I want to keep my kids cavity-free.

This is a guide designed to be practical, not drive you crazy, and to keep your child healthy, and away from the needle and drill—with the least amount of effort possible.

It does take some changes, but it is most likely not what you were expecting. It is what I do to keep my own kids cavity-free and how I have already helped thousands of families in my own practice. It will help your family as well.

I had one mom whose oldest son had eight cavities when we met five years ago. Now, the two younger siblings have zero cavities. Mom told me, "We did what you told us, Dr. Lucas. We threw out the crackers. We have ice cream most nights. We don't even floss, and our younger kids don't have cavities." I can't promise it will be that simple for everyone, (and I still recommend flossing), but I can show you why preventing cavities can actually be less work instead of more effort.

In similar fashion, some of my pediatric dental colleagues read my book before publication. One dentist (who shall remain nameless forever) told me he didn't agree with everything in my book. A few months later, he came back to me and said, "I apologize. I now agree with you. I just did my own children's exams and they both have cavities in between the teeth, even though we floss. I think you are on to something."

Hopefully you can change your dentist's mind and encourage them to focus more on diet for prevention, helping them be more effective with their prevention program. I will also show you why some otherwise healthy diets accidentally cause cavities and how to avoid it.

I have spent years researching scientific journals, examining chemical and microbiology reactions in textbooks, looking at the biochemistry, and thousands of families have used my methods with great results. The good news is that prevention takes less effort when you focus on diet.

The best time to read this is before your child is one year old. However, many of you will pick up this book because your child already "accidentally" had eight cavities, as is extremely common, and it will still be helpful to you for the future. Or perhaps you are curious in regards to your own dental health. It is never too late to switch to healthier habits for teeth. My principles apply to teenagers and adults as well, although I write it from the perspective of being a parent.

No, I am not going to tell you to give your kids chocolate all day, but I will tell you why I give my kids both dark chocolate and ice cream more than any other dentist would recommend, and why it makes sense from a biochemistry perspective.

Introduction

As a pediatric dentist, I have permanent job security because, according to the most recent reports by the American Academy of Pediatric Dentistry (AAPD), over 60 percent of children in America have a cavity by age five. But I also have a heart—and three little daughters of my own whom I want to keep cavity-free. Seeing the dental destruction in the mouths of far too many children and the tears that often come as I repair children's teeth have kept me searching for better ways to prevent the cavities that plague children (and adults too).

Most parents are surprised when their children get cavities. The dentist told them that if they brushed long enough, got enough fluoride, and didn't eat too much candy or drink any soda, that would be enough to prevent cavities. In fact, many dentists, doctors, and nutritionists have children with cavities and no idea how they got there.

So when cavities formed, as they inevitably do, all a dentist could say (until now) was that "some kids have weak teeth." But the true cause of cavities is simple, and once you understand it, cavities don't have to be an unavoidable given for you or your child. As we go forward in this book, I'll explain how easy it is to get cavities without ever touching candy or soda. And I'll also explain how easy it is to prevent cavities, because keeping your primary (baby) teeth is very important.

My goal is that you find this book so refreshingly helpful that you will want to give copies to your parent friends and even your dentist. My goal is to change the paradigm on how the world thinks about cavity prevention by making it simpler, and focusing on diet first. This book can save you decades of hopeless frustration at the dental office.

Here is what Erin, a mother of five, said after reading this book:

> "I must say, I definitely wish I had known this stuff years ago, before a majority of my kids grew up. But, alas, my youngest is just one year old and will benefit greatly from you sharing your knowledge. I love your writing style. As a mother of five, I could personally relate to every example you gave, and I felt you were writing this book for parents out of genuine concern and with no condemnation. I also thought it was a nice touch that

you mentioned what you make for your family at home as a father and not just a dentist.

"Personally, I feel this book should sit on the shelves right next to *What to Expect When You are Expecting*. The lessons are invaluable, and, as you mention more than once, it starts by age one."

WHY PREVENTION IS IMPORTANT: BABY TEETH STORIES

The best way to explain the importance of prevention is to review a few scenarios that I commonly see. These scenarios happen in dental offices across the country every day.

Scenario 1

You confidently bring your five-year-old son in for his regular dental exam. You have been very attentive to his dental health, bringing him in every six months. You spend a lot of time brushing his teeth before bed. Of course he has the occasional piece of candy, but definitely not every day. He drinks juice only at breakfast. Soda is not allowed in the house. While the dental assistant cleans his teeth, she comments on how healthy his gums look and what a great job of brushing you are doing. As she takes his first-ever x-rays, you are feeling great and just a tiny bit superior to the other parents who give their kids junk food all the time. Although you know you are not perfect, you are trying very hard to do what is right for your child.

Next, the dentist returns with the x-rays and says, "Your son has eight cavities and needs eight fillings."

Your jaw drops, and you enter the stages of cavity-grief: denial, anger, fear, and guilt.

Stage one: denial. How can this be? You ask the dentist if she is sure. She shows you the dark spots on the x-rays; the cavities are clearly visible. Quickly, you move to the second stage: anger. What have all the checkups and fluoride treatments been for? My kid doesn't even have soda. We barely have candy. We don't deserve this!

After the anger subsides a little, you realize that these are only baby teeth, and you wait for the dentist to tell you this. You want to hurry this process along, so you ask, "But these are just baby teeth. They are going to fall out anyway, so we don't have to fix them, right?"

Your dentist responds, "Yes, these teeth do fall out, but, unfortunately, not for another five to seven years."

You think, *Five to seven years! I remember losing my baby teeth around age six. I swear I was in kindergarten. I don't remember losing any when I was ten. Maybe I should Google this. Surely the dentist is confused.* Then the dentist explains that children lose their front baby teeth early but don't lose the back ones until much later. It's then that you have a vague memory of tossing a freshly lost baby tooth onto the soccer field during practice once, but it's very hazy.

Now, the next stage sets in: fear. You remember absolutely *hating* the dentist when you were a child. You *still* don't like going. In fact, you bring your kids to the dentist more often than you go for yourself because you wanted to avoid the awful drill-and-fill experience for them. You've done everything in your power to prevent this. You've been so conscientious, trying *so hard* for this to not happen. Of course you haven't been perfect, but you felt really darn close.

Next stage: guilt. This overwhelming sensation of guilt may or may not have started upon first learning of the eight cavities, but it certainly follows fear. You're thinking, *Only bad parents let their kids get eight cavities!* You obviously missed something. At this point you don't yet know that a majority of children in America get at least one cavity and that the typical pattern is to get eight of them (and most are not caused by eating candy). Even if you knew that, it wouldn't make you feel any better. And right now, your biggest concern is how your son will fare with the needles and the drill.

Scenario 2

The following scenario happens less often, but for the parents who do experience it, it is not something they wished for.

You bring your two-year-old son into the office for his first checkup. Your family doctor and family dentist (both of whom you have been seeing for decades) said you didn't need to bring him in until age three. But you have noticed a few dark spots on his front teeth, and you are worried they are cavities. Your child doesn't even know what candy is, so you consider this odd. You're not too worried, though, because they're just baby teeth. But you don't like how the brown spots look.

Once in the exam room, you try to coax your boy into the exam chair, but it doesn't work, which you had kind of figured since your son cries when he gets his hair cut or his ears checked. The dentist does a brief visual exam of your son's teeth with your son in your lap.

The dentist confirms your fears that the brown spots indeed are cavities and then gives you two heart-wrenching options, neither of which you are prepared for. You can save the teeth so that they look better until age six or seven, when they will naturally fall out, or take a wait-and-see approach until your son is older. However, if you wait, it is likely that the cavities will grow, forcing you to have the teeth extracted at some point. Depending on when the teeth are pulled, your child may be without front teeth for a few years. The dentist then explains that if you decide to fix the teeth now, your son needs to have very deep sedation (general anesthesia) for the procedure because of his age. The bill for this is in the thousands of dollars instead of in the hundreds. Additionally, if you wait, there is no way to predict whether your child will need the expensive sedation or not when the time comes to treat the teeth. It is perhaps possible to prevent the cavities from growing, but this is much more difficult than preventing cavities in the first place.

So you're left with the awful predicament of paying thousands of dollars to save your child's teeth now and sedating him or her to do so, or of waiting to see if they will need to be extracted later, potentially leaving the child with missing front teeth for a few years. Wouldn't it be nice to avoid this difficult decision in the first place? This is a discussion I wish never to have to have with parents again. If you start thinking about prevention correctly at age one, it is completely preventable.

WHO THIS BOOK IS FOR

This book is *not* for parents who need motivation to cut back on soda or candy for their children. I assume everyone who reads this book already understands this basic concept. In fact, if I mention sweets in this book, it is to tell you which ones I recommend. I have seen hundreds of parents try to avoid all sugar and still accidentally give their child cavities. This book is intended for parents who are motivated to keep their children cavity-free and not be accidentally surprised, as millions of parents have been for generations before them.

Your motivation is likely one of the following. You may simply want to avoid needles, drills, and pain for your child because you were afraid of the dentist. You may want a healthy mouth for your child. You may want to avoid your child needing teeth extracted early because of cavities and then having spacing issues in his or her adult teeth. You may want to know how to prevent your child from having eight cavities. You may be thrifty and want to save money at the dentist. No matter what your motivation, this book can help you.

This book is for all parents who want their children to be cavity-free, in the easiest way possible, thereby avoiding the consequent fillings that cavities require. However, it is also for parents who want to prevent their children from having eight cavities when they're only five years old or younger. The way cavities work is that they often form on all of the back teeth at the same time. It's often, unfortunately, an all-or-nothing situation. So, whether your goal is dental perfection or simply to avoid "cavity disaster," this book is for you. What you may find, however, is that even if you are simply trying to avoid a cavity disaster with your child, by following the advice I present in this book, your child may end up with zero cavities—without you even trying that hard. If you want to learn from the accidental "cavity mistakes" and "cavity successes" of other families that have gone before you, I have taken the experiences of thousands of families and analyzed them for you, added in my dental-biochemistry background, and simplified it for you as a set of principles, tips, and motivational tricks to succeed.

The good news is that it is easier than you think, if you focus on the principles in my book. My advice is also completely different from what you expect to hear. It's practical, real-life advice. My goal is to expend the least amount of energy as possible and still have complete success. Not everyone will agree with everything I have to say—but it works because it is based on mathematics.

WHY SHOULD YOU LISTEN TO ME?

I am a board-certified pediatric dentist who has performed more than twenty thousand dental exams. I see more children in a year than most general dentists see in ten years. I have won the Seattle-area ParentMap's Pediatric Dentist Golden Teddy award for five years in a row. But that isn't all that gives me expertise in solving the cavity riddle; I also have a biochemistry background and believe that mathematics can explain everything in the universe. Biochemists have to know and understand all the biological and chemical processes of living things (including how food breaks down). In fact, many of the current popular books regarding nutrition are written by biochemists like me.

With that biochem background and so much experience under my belt—and with the dental health of my patients and my own daughters at stake—I decided to try to solve the riddle of exactly how cavities form. The answers I'd been given in dental school didn't suffice, so I started digging into the biochemical and biological sciences. What I developed is a zero-cavities program for our children that includes more chocolate and ice cream and less fluoride, and it eliminates the drawn-out tooth-brushing torture (only twenty seconds' worth instead of two minutes for very young children). It all comes down to simple biochemistry and math.

My principles have been tested on my patients over the last four years. I am blessed to have a patient base of over three thousand active patients. I have countless families who came to me originally, years ago, because their oldest child had a mouthful of cavities. Years later, their younger children are cavity-free because they applied what I taught them. If it were only up to genetics, this would never happen. Of course, the parents made the decision to switch to healthy habits themselves. I can't take all of the credit. I have been much more fulfilled as a dentist knowing that I can make a difference in children's lives instead of saying, "It's just weak enamel. There is nothing you can do." I have learned so much from the wonderful families in my office and am passing that information on to you. Everything you learn from me was taught to me by another parent.

CAVITIES ARE LIKE FINANCES

The way to get zero cavities is so simple, you may feel like Dorothy from *The Wizard of Oz*—you had the power all along, but no one ever told you that simply tapping your ruby slippers together was the secret. However, like many things in life, just because something is simple, that doesn't necessarily make it easy or intuitive. Preventing cavities is similar to keeping your finances in order. Both take years of practicing habits before there are any consequences, good or bad. There is no immediate feedback. Similar to bad debt, cavities can sometimes take years to develop before they are noticed. A financial guru could simply tell you, "Don't go into credit-card debt," but that wouldn't be that helpful. Understanding the habits needed for and the psychology about controlling your finances, as well as setting up good systems, makes you more likely to be successful. Just ask Dave Ramsey, the personal finance guru. In the same way, I won't simply tell you, "Avoid all starches." Similar to a book on personal finances, most of this book is about the psychology of setting up good habits and setting yourself up for success. Of course, it doesn't hurt that I have a view on cavity prevention that is focused more on diet than is the current dogma. Additionally, understanding the reasoning behind my principles will help you implement them better in the long term. When the next new food fad comes out, you can take what you've learned and apply it. The groceries at the warehouse stores will change over the years, but the way cavities work isn't changing anytime soon. I hope, however, that the way you think about cavities will be changed by the time you finish this book.

GUIDE TO READING THIS BOOK

This book is split into four different parts. Part I explains why baby teeth are important. Part II explains the underlying mechanism of cavity formation, so you know why it works. Part III explains my three prevention principles and gives tips about how to employ them at different ages and stages. Part IV discusses frequently asked questions and other miscellaneous pediatric dentistry topics.

Being a parent of three myself, I realize that you will read this book the way I read parenting books: skipping chapters that don't apply to you. Please do exactly this. Skim, and skip ahead as you see fit. When my oldest child was an infant, I read four different books about sleep, all recommending contradictory advice, and I never finished a single one, even if I appreciated them all. All of my chapters are important, but some of them may be more important to you right now than others. That is OK.

I will say this: Make sure you read the chapters "The Math of Cavity Formation" and "Emotional Intelligence and Cavity Prevention." Preventing cavities is mathematical yet very emotional, so those are the two most important chapters in addition to the basic principles.

Some of my most helpful items are lists and graphics, most of which can be downloaded (and printed out) from TheDentistDad.com. Feel free to e-mail me via the TheDentistDad.com. If you send me a message, I will do my best to respond.

If you are a dentist and think this book would be helpful for your patients, contact me via TheDentistDad.com/dentists for information on free handouts for patients and discounted copies with zero hassle. As dentists, we should be leading the diet-based prevention approach, not shying away from it.

Terminology: *Cavitation caused by dental caries* is the technically correct term for the bacterial disease process that produces a cavity. I have intentionally used the term *cavity* or *cavities* instead of *cavitation* or *caries* to make this book more reader friendly.

Pronouns: In my practice we see every combination of families with children: moms, dads, grandparents, adoptive parents, guardians, and beyond. When referring to parents, I refer to mom and dad arbitrarily, but realize that any parent or guardian combination can be substituted at any time. Instead of saying "either mom or dad or parent" every time, my editor and I arbitrarily chose to randomly select a pronoun so the sentences flow more smoothly with an active voice.

Remember: There is never a guarantee of a desired outcome when it comes to health or oral health. In science, everything is a hypothesis. My goal is to change the type of research that is done to focus more on diet, but there is always more research to be done. Please bring your child to a dentist at age one and follow his or her advice.

Part I

The Three Most Common Myths
About Cavities In Baby Teeth

As we begin, let me explain briefly the three most common myths about cavities in baby teeth. Then I will address each myth individually in more depth later.

Myth 1: You lose your baby teeth at age six, so they don't matter.

This is the easiest to address since it is really just a misconception, not a myth. You don't lose your back baby molars until between ten and twelve years of age, so if you have a hole in your molar at age five, you don't want to just "yank it out." That was an easy one.

Myth 2: Cavities are mostly caused by genetics—whether you have strong or weak enamel—so there is not too much you can do to prevent them.

While genetics play a role in everything, cavities in your child are 95 to 100 percent preventable if you know exactly what to do and start thinking with the mind-set that diet causes cavities. Genetics are correlated with cavities but do not cause cavities. Diet causes cavities. Obviously, some parents will have to try harder than others because of genetics, but that doesn't mean it's not possible. Successful people focus only on what they have control over. When it comes down to it, it doesn't matter how much genetics plays a role, because you have no control over it. Focus only on the things you have control over. This is true in life and in cavity prevention. We should keep studying genetics in dentistry to look for breakthroughs, but that isn't going to help you keep your child cavity-free right now.

Myth 3: If I don't give my kids candy or soda—or even juice—and I brush their teeth really well, they won't get cavities.

This is the biggest myth that needs to be debunked. Before I recognized the true cause of cavities, I always had some patients whose parents would end up surprised when the child had eight cavities by age five even though the parents were doing all of the "traditional" prevention techniques (not eating much candy, brushing for two minutes every night, not drinking juice all day long). These kids had cavities that fell into the "unexplained" category or would be blamed on weak enamel. Their parents were trying extra hard but were still ending up with results opposite of what they expected. Obviously, if you give your children soda or candy all the time, they will likely get cavities faster than a speeding bullet. Most parents are not doing this, yet 60 percent of five-year-olds still have cavities.

Let's address myth #1 first – why baby teeth matter.

BUT THEY'RE JUST BABY TEETH; WHY FIX THEM?

When parents discover that their children's primary teeth need work, they always ask, "But aren't they just baby teeth?" Once you know why baby teeth are important, you will understand the need for cavity prevention from the moment teeth come in.

Children develop twenty baby teeth. The earliest erupt (come in) between three and nine months of age, and the last ones usually between two and three years of age. The front teeth (incisors) are the ones that are the most celebrated and memorable, and they are also the first to fall out. When they fall out between six and eight years of age, they are commemorated with pictures, videos, and visits by the tooth fairy. But what if your child gets a cavity in a front tooth at age three? Cavities can cause pain and sensitivity and distract children at preschool or kindergarten. Most children this age won't be able to verbalize that their teeth are sensitive, so it is easy for it to go unnoticed. If the tooth does get pulled out, your child will be missing it for three to ten years.

Many two- and three-year-olds get cavities. In fact, the incidence of cavities in preschool children has actually increased over the past thirty years despite decreasing in every other demographic. But if enough parents, health-care providers, and caregivers learn the principles in this book, this trend can be reversed. We need to think about preventing cavities at age one if we want to prevent our three-year-olds from going through painful treatment procedures (in most cases small children require either surgery or moderate oral sedation).

The back (posterior) baby teeth—the canines and molars—I call the "forgotten baby teeth." By the time they come in, parents are relieved that teething is over, and nobody remembers when those teeth fall out. But those primary molars remain in place until ten to twelve years of age. Some children get them in at eighteen months, and almost all children have some, if not all, of them by age two. So parents have to take care of their kids' molars for eight to ten years! If the molars are neglected enough to require extraction (because of a lack of dental knowledge), the child doesn't have a tooth to chew on for up to a decade!

If for some reason you still are not convinced that chewing or avoiding pain is important, then you should at least care about your child's adult teeth. Getting an infection in a baby tooth at an early age can damage the developing adult tooth. Additionally, if you have to extract a baby molar too early, you may lose space for the permanent teeth that come in years later. This could require more extensive orthodontic treatment to make room for the adult teeth, or, in extreme cases, the extraction of a perfectly good adult tooth.

PROACTIVE PREVENTION INSTEAD OF REACTIVE REPAIRS

For many years, dentistry has been reactive. Dentists drill and fill cavities that form. However, if we want to see a large decrease in cavities, dentists everywhere need to be more proactive and start acknowledging that cavities are indeed 95–100 percent preventable with dietary changes.

Current thinking is that some children have weak enamel and that there is not much they can do to prevent cavities from forming. But do 60 percent of children under five really have weak enamel? No! The reality is only about 1–3 percent of the population has some true genetic mutation or developmental defect in their enamel. The problem is that diet trumps most everything else in cavity formation and prevention, but that is not how dentists are classically trained. In dental school, it is genetics first, then fluoride, and then diet. As I will show you, diet should come first. What dentists are currently taught still works, of course, but diet is most important. Fluoride can help reduce cavities by about 20–30 percent. Genetics can sway things by a variable number of percentage points. For a 98 percent reduction in cavities, focus on diet.

Obviously, there is a genetic component, and some children (and adults) are more or less prone to cavities than others. But cavities are still caused by the same bacteriological process. If you have genetically strong teeth and you do the opposite of my three prevention principles, your genetics won't matter. If you are more prone to cavities, you may have to do more than average, but cavity prevention is still possible.

The reason my three prevention principles are so revolutionary is that they are a *practical* way to prevent cavities by focusing less on brushing or flossing and more on snack foods. Being a dentist who says diet is more important than everything else is an alternative view, but it shouldn't be. However, instead of offering an impractical diet approach, such as strict paleo or all raw foods, I can tell you exactly where you can cheat and where you can't. It is important to know where you can be imperfect, especially while raising young children.

As for brushing, the current brush-for-two-minutes advice is impractical for very young children—plus, it doesn't work on them. While I support the idea of brushing a seven-year-old's teeth for two minutes twice a day (even though I personally rarely make it that long) you can't use the same advice for a one-, two-, or three-year-old and expect parents to do it. Has anyone making these recommendations actually spent two minutes twice a day brushing an uncooperative two-year-old's teeth? Brushing that way won't change anything in that age category if you don't focus on diet. Of course, brushing is still a requirement for cavity prevention, but if you focus on dietary changes first, you will realize that you can shorten brushing from two minutes for very young children and still end up with zero cavities.

The great thing about my principles is that if you start thinking about them when your child is a one-year-old, it will actually be *less* work to instill cavity-preventing habits than cavity-causing habits. This is because it is easier to *start* a habit than it is to *change* a habit.

Note: While prevention is always the ideal goal, keep in mind that if a child comes for his or her first visit with eight cavities, I sometimes make a special effort to *not* talk about prevention, and your dentist may do the same. We have already missed the prevention window, and dentists are compassionate people. We don't look for ways to make parents feel guilty. We fix the teeth, and then later we gingerly discuss prevention.

CAN'T WE JUST FIX THEM?

By now, I have made the argument of why baby teeth are important to fix if they have a hole in them. Can't we just fix cavities in today's modern age and move on? Of course we can. But that isn't always a perfect solution. As a pediatric dentist who has worked with thousands of children who are either sensitive, strong-willed, have a strong gag reflex, hyperactive, ASD, or have a history of negative experiences at a previous dentist, I have learned one thing: it is impossible to always predict how a particular child will act after giving them an injection and trying to drill out a cavity. Also, since children will often get eight cavities at the same time, it is much more uncomfortable to fix eight cavities than zero, no matter how well-behaved a preschooler or kindergartener may be. As soon as I start to think that I can manage any child's behavior perfectly, I am humbled by a four-year-old who walks in the door. Even if a pediatric dentist is able to treat 95% of patients with superior behavior management skills, there will always be 5% who are going to have a bad time. Let me give you a few different reasons why you would want to avoid having to fix cavities, if you weren't convinced already:

1) Your child is more anxious or sensitive, and might happen to be in the 5% of children who comes away with a negative experience (even if 95% of other children do well).

2) Having a phobia of the dentist is usually on any person's top five list of fears, right up there with public speaking and death. Avoiding fillings and extractions is the easiest way to prevent this fear of discomfort.

3) If your child happens to not be able to cooperate for multiple appointments at age four or five, then the fillings may require more invasive sedation or surgery.

4) From a natural point of view: in an ideal world, we would like to keep our teeth intact, and not fill them with any foreign substance.

BABY TEETH SUMMARY

Society as a whole needs to start realizing the importance of baby teeth. Right now, most parents become aware of how important baby teeth are only after there is a need to fix them. And it's not only parents. Many general dentists and well-meaning physicians don't have a healthy respect for the primary dentition, as evidenced by their instructing parents to take a child to the dentist at three or four years of age, which leads to reactive rather than proactive care. Of course, if the dentist or doctor does not know about proactive pediatric cavity prevention, he or she won't realize how helpful visiting early would be.

If your dentist doesn't believe diet is the most important thing in cavity prevention, don't hold it against him.

This does not discredit the other things he has to say about prevention. Simply give him or her a copy of this book. Direct them to TheDentistDad.com/dentists for contact information.

Now that you know about the importance of maintaining baby teeth, let's talk about the cavity process itself so we can better understand how to stop it.

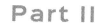

Part II

How Cavities Are Formed

Although I will share some technical information in this section, once you understand the underlying process of how cavities form, you will know exactly why my three principles of prevention are so effective and why little cavities matter too. Then you'll be better able to master the principles and remember them forever. You will also understand why a problem as complex as cavities can be prevented with three relatively simple principles.

THE REAL CAUSE OF CAVITIES

When we talk about cavities, what we are really talking about is a bacterial disease. Cavities are the result of a disease process called "caries," which is caused by specific bacteria. In dental school, our instructors hammered into us that "caries is a process," but it took me years of staring at teeth to realize what they actually meant. Here's the broad outline; then we'll go into more detail.

1. Bacteria live in the mouth and grow on teeth.
2. Mouth bacteria break down simple carbohydrates into lactic acid as part of digestion.
3. If enough lactic acid sits on a tooth for long enough, it dissolves part of the tooth and forms a hole in the tooth.

This hole is called a cavity. To prevent cavities, you need a strategy to interrupt this cycle.

A cavity does not form with one cycle. It happens over hundreds, more likely thousands, of cycles. You will not get cavities from snacking on treats in one weekend at Grandma's house or from a few days at Disneyland. You get them from your everyday habits repeated 365 days a year. If a habit is done three times a day, that is already 1,095 occurrences in a year. From ages two to five years, that is 3,285 times.

The math multiplies quickly. That is why dealing with this process (or at least thinking about it) by age one is so important. By age two, the habits you have started are already ingrained and most likely will stay the same or get worse over the next three years.

BACTERIA IS THE KEY TO UNDERSTANDING CAVITY FORMATION

When you focus on the simplest explanation for cavities, the most effective prevention strategies become more obvious. Let's look at the cavity cycle in more detail, so that the strategies I offer will make more sense.

1. Bacteria grow on teeth, forming plaque. Plaque is an accumulation of a lot of bacteria and biofilm (the goop that makes bacteria stick to teeth). Research shows that it takes about twenty-four hours for bacteria to form plaque. The most obvious prevention methods to lessen plaque are brushing and flossing. The fancy term for this is "oral hygiene."

2. Bacteria break down large quantities of simple carbohydrates into lactic acid, similar to how our muscles produce lactic acid when we work out. The same bacteria that break down glucose (or sucrose, or lactose, or anything that ends with "ose") also cause cavities when they produce enough lactic acid.

3. Lactic acid is one of the bacterial waste products produced when simple carbohydrates are converted into energy; it creates an environment in the mouth that is acidic enough to demineralize (dissolve) enamel if it sits on the tooth for long enough. Once the bacterial waste gets busy dissolving enamel, saliva comes to the rescue. But it takes about twenty minutes for saliva to rinse the mouth enough to reduce the acidity to stop the cavity-forming process.

4. Under normal circumstances, saliva remineralizes the tooth so that the hole is "patched up" by carrying minerals to it. This takes much longer. Let's estimate about two to three hours.

LACTIC ACID: THE GREAT DESTROYER

Most people know that you don't want to mess with acid. It burns and dissolves things, even in microscopic amounts. Enamel—the strongest component in the whole body—is actually dissolved by teeny-tiny bacterial waste in the form of lactic acid. So if you never brush your child's teeth in the correct way, millions of microscopic bacteria synergistically work together to create a complex enamel-destroying organism.

However, when simple carbohydrate concentrations are low, bacteria don't produce lactic acid. It's only produced from *large concentrations of simple carbohydrates* all at once. And without the lactic acid in the mouth, cavities will not form. Obviously then, the easiest way to stop the cavity process is to not let simple carbohydrates pass over the teeth constantly or let them sit on the teeth for very long. Take broccoli, for example: Although broccoli contains carbohydrates, the concentration of carbohydrates is relatively low compared with the water and fiber concentration, so it does not have a high enough concentration of carbohydrates for bacteria to make acid. Another way to say this is, simply, low-carb foods don't cause cavities. This explains why meat, nuts, cheese, and broccoli do not cause cavities. Protein and fat are different molecules from carbohydrates, so bacteria can still use them for energy, but they do not produce lactic acid when supplied with protein or fat.

Why does concentration of carbohydrates matter? The answer is pH. The term "pH" is an abbreviation for the concentration of acid or base molecules floating in water. The pH scale ranges from 0-14. A pH of 7 is neutral (drinking water). Acids have lower pH (more acid molecules), while bases have higher pH (more base molecules). Enamel (the outer layer of tooth) only dissolves with a pH below 5.5. So, if you don't get enough acid molecules to reach 5.5, enamel will not dissolve. If you don't have a high concentration of carbohydrates, the bacteria will never make enough lactic acid to reach the 5.5 pH threshold. This explains why raw kale or celery won't cause cavities. The low concentration of carbohydrates they contain will lower the pH slightly, but won't break the 5.5 barrier. A pH of 6.0 is still okay for enamel. Just don't convert the kale or celery into juice. This changes the properties of the carbohydrates. Also keep in mind that both citrus fruits and soda are very acidic, so don't have either in excess.

You could make the argument to switch to a low-carb diet for kids, but I would argue that is not practical. Also, fruits and vegetables are loaded with important vitamins and phytonutrients. As busy parents living in modern society, we need a practical solution. Since we aren't cutting out carbs anytime soon, does this mean we should brush after every meal? Although this is conventional wisdom, a much simpler approach that I propose is to simply choose foods that don't stick to teeth as long (such as a crunchy apple). Because carbohydrates are the only things that produce lactic acid, the most important variables to consider when preventing cavities are the frequency of carbohydrates and the stickiness of the carbohydrates.

Let's review:

1. Bacteria produce lactic acid only with a large quantity of carbohydrates.
2. Acid stays on the teeth for about twenty minutes.
3. Limiting the frequency of carbohydrates and stickiness of carbohydrates is more important than any other variable

We can survive without carbohydrates through a process called ketoacidosis. However, I wouldn't recommend cutting out carbohydrates for kids, because they are growing rapidly and their metabolisms are much faster than adults. So how is it possible to not get cavities if we eat carbohydrates? Part of the answer is the amount of time food stays on the teeth. The other part of the answer is equilibrium, which we will explain in the next chapter.

EQUILIBRIUM EXPLAINED (OR WHY OUR TEETH DON'T SPONTANEOUSLY FALL APART)

Equilibrium, in the context of teeth, means there is no net change in the amount of tooth structure over time; everything remains in balance. Another term for this is homeostasis. When we observe a tooth with our eyes over a period of an hour, it looks as if nothing is happening. But a lot is actually happening at a microscopic level.

Let's look at the example of drinking juice. When juice goes into your mouth, microscopic bacteria immediately begin processing the sugar (simple carbohydrates) into energy and lactic acid. The energy is then used to produce more bacteria. Once the acid is produced, it falls onto the tooth, dissolving a specific microscopic spot. If nothing happens from this point forward, those particular molecules of the tooth are gone forever and a microscopic hole develops.

When that microscopic process happens thousands of times, you get a macroscopic-size cavity visible to the naked eye (or an x-ray). Thankfully, however, with normal biology, something does happen. Saliva arrives to save the day.

Saliva serves the important purpose of rinsing away acid and remineralizing the tooth with calcium and phosphate. These vital minerals repair those damaged molecules and patch the microscopic hole back up. If a tooth is in equilibrium, the rate at which it dissolves and the rate at which it is remineralized are equal so that there is no net change to the tooth over time. If a tooth demineralizes at a rate faster than saliva can remineralize it, then equilibrium is lost. The tooth keeps dissolving over days and years until a cavity forms.

It all comes back to the twenty critical minutes it takes for saliva to do its job. For example, when you eat an apple, your teeth don't automatically fall apart because

the sugar from the apple does not overwhelm the heal-
ing power of saliva as long as you eat it as a snack once
a day. Water also rinses away acid. So if you simply have
your child sip on water after every snack or meal, this
alone should significantly reduce the potential for cavities. Keep in mind that water will rinse away acid, but it
won't rinse away sticky starches. Eating sticky starches
can actually be worse than sugar in some cases because
it doesn't rinse away as quickly.

Considering the fact that saliva is remineralizing, cavities are caused by reducing the amount of time teeth
spend in contact with saliva and increasing the amount
of time spent in contact with acid. Conversely, cavities
are prevented by decreasing the time a tooth spends in
contact with acid and increasing the time spent in contact with saliva. It really is that simple.

Remember that not all foods are created equal.
Some foods create lactic acid more easily than do others. Foods high in protein or fat (such as chicken, cheese,
or peanuts) will not create enough of a sugar spike in
one's mouth to form lactic acid. The mouth bacteria can
still convert protein and fat into carbohydrates to use
as energy, but the process is so slow that it doesn't produce lactic acid. Essentially, it is impossible to get cavities from eating protein or fat.

Conclusion: the amount of time teeth are exposed
to carbohydrates is the single most important factor in

cavity formation. Reduce the amount of time your child's teeth are exposed to carbohydrates and lactic acid, and you will reduce the chance for cavities. Choose unprocessed foods that take more time to break down and convert into energy; choose foods higher in protein and fats to reduce the mouth's acidic cavity-causing environment. When you do occasionally give your child food that is rich in carbohydrates, make sure it is a food that won't stay stuck on or in between the teeth for more than a minute. And help your saliva with a good rinse after eating.

This explains why teenagers who eat pizza and hamburgers and chug sodas down quickly (but not all day) somehow get zero cavities even though they are horrible brushers. With dramatic irony in full effect, the teenager who flosses every night and spends an inordinate amount of time brushing but slowly nibbles on pretzels all day and eats breakfast cereal for breakfast and dinner (another sticky starch) will be frustrated with cavities.

Cavities aren't fair. They play by different rules. Cavities only care about carbohydrates and time.

PROGRESSION OF CAVITIES

Cavities aren't born overnight. The bacteriological process that creates them takes time. But once the bacteria bore through the outer enamel, they continue through the inner dentin, and, if left untreated, will eat into the soft pulp of the tooth, where they cause infection. So the main reason we fix cavities is to prevent infection and pain. If cavities didn't cause infection, they wouldn't be a big deal.

Tooth pain for any length of time causes adults to seek treatment. But children sometimes experience only mild pain, and, often, they then get used to it, so they don't complain. I have had many parents report that their children became better eaters after we fixed their severe cavities because eating didn't hurt anymore.

Although most tooth infections are minor, some can be serious enough to cause swelling in the face. I see children with swollen faces in my practice a few times every year (and they are almost always patients whom I've never met before). These kinds of infections are usually resolved with antibiotics and extraction. Unfortunately, extracting an infected baby tooth is the most painful dental procedure a child can go through, and it dramatically lessens the chance of a positive experience at the dentist.

Left untreated, however, a severe infection in a baby tooth not only causes extreme pain, it can even lead to death. It doesn't happen very often, but the most recent publicized case was in Maryland in 2007 when a twelve-year-old boy died from an infection in a baby tooth.

Therefore, we fix the little cavities so they don't turn into medium-size cavities. We fix the medium-size cavities so they don't turn into large cavities. We fix the large cavities so they don't turn into an infection and pain. By the law of transition, we fix little cavities so that, ultimately, they don't turn into infection. (But with really little cavities in baby teeth, we often just monitor them and try to prevent them from growing.)

TREATMENT OPTIONS
There are multiple treatment options for primary teeth, and you can avoid them by preventing cavities. Treatment options include things called fillings, extractions, stainless steel crowns, pulpotomies, pulpectomies, space maintainers, oral sedation, general anesthesia, behavior management, and more. Discussing those treatment options is the subject of another book (probably a textbook). Realize that you can avoid what everyone else has to go through by preventing cavities.

Now, let's debunk Myth 2: Cavities are mostly caused by genetics—whether you have strong or weak enamel—so there is not too much you can do to prevent them.

WHY IT IS NOT JUST GENETICS
When I mention to people that I am writing a book about how to be cavity-free, they will either say, "I am blessed

with strong teeth, but my spouse is not so lucky," or they will ask, "Aren't cavities mostly genetics?"

The "old way" of thinking relies on the premise that cavities are caused by genetics or weak enamel, so other than brushing and flossing, using fluoride, and avoiding soda and candy, there is nothing you can do. This has been the way to explain cavity formation for those who keep getting cavities every few years despite their best efforts at prevention. If they've done the basics and still get cavities, these folks are simply told they have weak enamel. If you don't floss but don't have cavities, you must have strong enamel, or so the current dogma goes.

My research points to a new way of thinking that hypothesizes that the main cause of cavities is diet—specifically, easily digestible carbohydrates—and it explains a source of cavities that was once inexplicable. Starches, including not only sugar but also all processed flours, cling to the teeth and are then broken down by bacteria that live in the mouth, creating an acidic environment. This acidic environment sets the stage for cavities.

Flour has gone under the radar in dental schools as one of the main cavity causers for too long. However, it should be obvious by now that a processed starch that sticks very well to the teeth can easily cause cavities. My hypothesis that crackers and other dry cereals cause a large percentage of cavities explains cavity formation in many adults and children who were previously told they had weak enamel. If you're one of them, now there actually *is* something that you can do beyond the normal recommendations to prevent cavities. All dentists know carbohydrates cause cavities, but many of us have turned a blind eye to flour for decades. My hope is that this is emphasized in dental schools more in the future.

With this new understanding, it makes sense that even if you have great genetics and the strongest teeth in the world, you will still get cavities if you expose your teeth to carbohydrate-rich foods that stick to your teeth (such as crackers or dry cereals) in the way a small child does—for four hours a day over two or three years.

Of course, genetics does play a role in the development of cavities. Similar to type 2 diabetes or obesity, some people are simply more genetically predisposed to forming cavities. But lifestyle choices also play a big role. Even so, there will always be two children who do exactly the same thing, and one will be more prone to cavities. Some people will have to do more prevention and some less, but that doesn't change the fact that *the underlying cause of cavities is the natural bacterial process that breaks down the starches clinging to teeth*.

In books such as *Good Calories, Bad Calories*, by Gary Taubes, and *The Blood Sugar Solution*, and *Eat Fat, Get Thin* by Dr. Mark Hyman, a hypothesis is proposed that diabetes and obesity are also caused by the frequency of eating excess processed carbohydrates.

If you think about health with this newer hypothesis, then cavity prevention, diabetes, and obesity can all be prevented through reducing the frequency of blood sugar spikes. Dr. Philippe Hujoel, a professor from the University of Washington, wrote about this overall view on nutrition in relation to dental health back in 2009. For your body, insulin is the culprit. For your teeth, lactic acid is the culprit. I won't go into any more details with overall health, but I would recommend these books if you want to see nutrition views that don't blame genetics for everything. My recommendations take a more practical approach for children, so we don't get as idealistic as these other nutrition programs. From my experience, switching to a whole foods diet is much more difficult when you have children under five years old. As a rule, however, the more whole food, the better.

WHAT AGE THE TEETH TOUCH IS IMPORTANT

One of the most obvious genetic factors affecting the development of cavities in children is the age at which a child's teeth start to touch. For example, if the front top two teeth start touching each other at age one, a child is more likely to get a cavity—with everything else being equal—in between those teeth by age three. The parent of such a child would have to do more prevention work such as floss that one spot a few nights a week or more aggressively cut out processed carbohydrates from the child's diet. Kids whose front top teeth do not touch might never floss before age three and still not get a cavity in between those teeth.

If the back molars start to touch at age two in one child while in another child they don't touch until age four, the child whose teeth started touching earlier will be exponentially more prone to cavities. The food will be getting stuck in between the teeth for two more years. When your child's back teeth start to touch is one of the genetic factors that you cannot control. It is completely true that if your child's back teeth touch at age two, you will have to give her a much more "tooth-friendly" diet compared with the diet you could give another child whose back teeth do not touch until, say, age four.

Genetics (as in crowded teeth versus teeth with lots of space) simply make it harder to prevent cavities for some and easier for others. If your child's teeth aren't touching at age four, sing hallelujah! The later, the luckier. Only a small percentage of children and parents are that lucky. However, genetics don't change the underlying process. I want to emphasize that even if your child's teeth are crowded, zero cavities are still possible. You will simply have to be more gung ho about it.

There is a small percentage of people who truly do have teeth with weak enamel and some teeth that fall apart no matter what. However, this is only 1–3 percent of the population, and, statistically speaking, it most likely does not apply to you. The rest of us have normal enamel and are simply getting cavities from eating processed carbohydrates too frequently throughout the day and letting them stay on our teeth.

The main hurdle for many people is to realize that processed flour can easily cause cavities. I contend that frequent, processed flour in a dry form (such as crackers or cereal) is the major culprit in cavity formation for those who have already cut out most sugars, especially for those whose teeth are more crowded.

Don't Worry

If you're getting worried, don't. The secret to zero cavities is not to cut out all processed flour. I promised this book would be practical, and it is. Thankfully, I am not worried about macaroni and cheese or spaghetti because soft pastas do not stay on teeth for long. And a vital factor in cavity formation is how long foods stay on the teeth. It's the processed flours in snack crackers that are the problem; they stick to the teeth in a way that pasta does not because they are dried. Every dentist knows that dried fruit should be eaten in moderation because it sticks to the teeth. Fresh fruit has the same amount of sugar but does not stick. If you think about it, crackers are just dried bread. Bread has the same amount of flour and starch as a cracker, but it does not stick to teeth as crackers do. The solution is simple. Eat bread and fresh fruit instead of crackers and dried fruit. Also, no kid (whom I know) eats bread or spaghetti all day long, so that alone makes it ten times better than crackers. Meals aren't the big problem. It's the snacking that worries me, and it should worry you.

THE MATH OF CAVITY FORMATION

While it is admittedly an oversimplification, cavity formation is a straightforward biochemical reaction that can be stated as a mathematical formula with three major variables. The variables are plaque thickness, concentration of easily digestible carbohydrates, and time. The most important variable is the amount of time the simple carbohydrates remain on the teeth. If you take out time or the simple carbohydrates, there is no cavity. To make an environment acidic, you need a lot of lactic acid produced in a short amount of time. Remember that bacteria produce lactic acid only when given carbohydrates. Therefore, if you don't give bacteria a large quantity of carbohydrates, they won't produce acid fast enough to make an acidic environment. You can limit the lactic acid, therefore, by either choosing foods that are low in carbohydrates (e.g., crunchy vegetables, meat, etc.) or strictly limiting the time the carbohydrates are on the teeth (e.g., smoothies and yogurt both have a ton of sugar but rinse from teeth quickly.) Bacteria can produce acid only while in contact with carbohydrates, and that acid lasts for twenty minutes. It really is that simple.

A group of Swedish researchers created a mathematical formula to calculate the rate of cavity formation, and it is surprisingly accurate. Their mathematical formulas matched up almost exactly with what has been shown in clinical studies for decades. Cavity formation can be explained by mathematics because it all goes back to inorganic chemistry equations of acid dissolving enamel. The constants for these equations are in college textbooks. This wasn't surprising. What was surprising was the conclusion that the *frequency* of simple carbohydrate consumption *is more important than the amount* consumed. Therefore, sipping on a soda for four hours is much worse than drinking it in ten minutes. Grazing on bite-size, sticky crackers for a couple of hours is much worse than eating a snack in ten minutes and rinsing with a drink of water afterward. Although the researchers use soda as an example, the same concept applies to other foods. It even applies to milk (a staple in the bottles and sippy cups of most toddlers). Drinking milk at a meal is not bad for your teeth, but sipping on milk for four hours is.

The bottom line? The longer a food or drink is on the teeth, the more likely it is that a cavity will form. In the Swedish calculations, the person who sipped on a soda over fifty minutes had more *than double the enamel demineralization* (dissolved enamel) than the person who chugged the soda in a few minutes. Many toddlers with sippy cups of juice or milk who sip throughout the day have the potential to *get cavities sixteen times faster* than the child who sips on water all day and only drinks milk with meals.

The biochemistry-based math formulas and all of the clinical studies from the last sixty years tell us the same thing: acid lasts about twenty minutes on the tooth after the carbohydrates go away. Time is the most important variable to focus on to prevent cavities. So it is easy to see why keeping snack times organized is vital to cavity prevention.

Water is a potent ally in cavity prevention because the adage "the solution to pollution is dilution" holds true. Drinking water with, or immediately after, meals and snacks is a simple way to reduce cavity worry. This is why I give my kids whole milk or water with meals. I try to limit them to one smoothie a day during a meal. Whole milk is better for teeth than juice during a meal because of the higher fat content.

CAVITIES ARE 100 PERCENT PREVENTABLE

Cavities are 100 percent preventable with diet. Let me repeat that. Cavities are 100 percent preventable.[1] This

---

1 This is not including the 1–3% of the population that has enamel hypoplasia or a rare genetic anomaly. However, cavities are still *theoretically* preventable through diet even with these conditions, although not in a practical sense because switching children to an extremely low-carbohydrate diet is not practical. So for individuals

is not what they teach in dental school—not yet, any-way. However, it is important that you understand this new approach so you can understand how to "work the system."

In dental school they teach that if you eat foods that break down into sugars, mouth bacteria produce lactic acid (which, as a reminder, starts the cavity-formation process). Carbohydrates always convert to sugars and are in everyone's diet; therefore, cavities are impossible to prevent by diet modification according to the old dogma.

This is not true because not all foods are equal. Certain foods, such as those comprised of protein or fat, or fibrous vegetables such as broccoli, don't have a car-bohydrate concentration high enough to produce lactic acid. Bacteria produce lactic acid only if they have *high* concentrations of *simple* carbohydrates, so foods with low concentrations won't produce cavities. Therefore, if you ate only chicken and raw broccoli, you would never even have to brush, and cavities would never occur.

Because it's such a bold statement, let me repeat that. If you ate only chicken and raw broccoli (hypothetically),

---

with truly weak enamel, preventing cavities is *theoretically*, but not practically, true, as it can be for individuals with normal enamel. This is getting into semantics somewhat, but my point is that cavities are caused by diet and are, therefore, preventable by diet. Children who can eat only through a g-tube, for example, never get cavities unless they start to eat food or drink by mouth.

you would not get any cavities. Even if you slacked on brushing and a lot of bacteria were hanging out, they still need the high concentrations of carbohydrates in order to make acid. Acid is what makes the cavity. Study after study shows that certain foods that are low in carbohydrate concentrations (such as meat, nuts, cheese, and broccoli) do not produce enough lactic acid from bacteria to dissolve enamel. Even though these low carbohydrate foods have been shown individually to not make enough acid for cavities, some dentists still do not believe diet is the most important thing in cavity prevention. Diet is indeed the secret to cavity prevention. Even though you are not going to cut out all carbohydrates—nor should you—it is critical to understand this concept because, eventually, you will eat some foods containing carbohydrates. Diet is the trump card for brushing and flossing. If you floss your child's teeth twice a day but let him drink chocolate milk all day long, your child will still get cavities. If you (theoretically) give your child no processed foods, only whole foods, and mostly low-carbohydrate snacks, you could never floss and still achieve zero cavities. This is not what is taught in dental schools, but it should be. Diet trumps brushing and flossing. You should still brush and floss because, for 99 percent of families with young children, going to a completely whole food, low-carbohydrate diet is unfortunately not happening anytime soon. However, realizing that low-carb foods and whole foods are better for your teeth puts you ahead of the curve in terms of understanding cavity prevention.

Even carbohydrate-rich foods won't necessarily produce cavities. A whole apple (high in carbs when compared with broccoli) technically is capable of causing a cavity, but in practice, it will not do so. Because an apple has fiber and fiber makes you feel full, an apple is self-limiting. It is the rare person who would eat an apple by slowly taking a bite every twenty minutes for five hours a day, every day for a year. Normal people don't graze on apples for long periods of time. So if you eat an apple once or twice a day, the sugar is only on your teeth for twenty to forty minutes. In fact, having an apple once or twice a day is *recommended* for your teeth because it is crunchy (and it means you are not eating something else that causes cavities faster). The more you chew crunchy fruits or vegetables, the more saliva that is made. The act of chewing stimulates saliva flow. But an apple five times a day would be less preferable than mixing things up with other snack categories, such as cheese, nuts, or crunchy vegetables.

As you can see, you don't have to eliminate all carbohydrates from the diet. You just have to change the quality of the carbohydrates and how they are consumed. If the carbohydrate is easy to digest (and therefore easily converted into lactic acid), it has the potential to cause cavities. If you make the bacteria work harder by including fiber and not processing it before it enters the mouth, they won't be able to make an acidic environment fast enough. Remember, bacteria have no arms or legs. The bacteria only eat what you give them. Cavity-causing bacteria prefer starches that stay close to them longer, since all of their food has to come to them. Ironically, sugars can rinse away from the teeth faster than many starches.

Let's debunk our final myth:

Myth 3: If I don't give my kids candy or soda—or even juice—and I brush their teeth really well, they won't get cavities.
By looking at the biochemistry of cavities, you will see why some otherwise very nutritious foods could accidentally cause cavities in your child and, more importantly, how to avoid the accidental cavities. There are many other hidden sources of simple carbohydrates that are just as important.

NOT ALL CARBS ARE EQUAL: THE BIOCHEMISTRY OF CAVITIES
Candy and soda are the most obvious forms of sugar. A less obvious form of sugar is processed flour (and all flour today is processed). Don't worry, though. My prevention

plan does not ban all flour, just crackers and flour cereals because they are dry. Understanding some details about carbohydrates will help you apply these concepts on your own, even without a list.

So to explain why carbohydrates like flour have more potential to cause cavities than other foods do, here's a quick biochemistry lesson about how a simple carbohydrate's molecular structure looks as compared with the complex structure of fats and proteins. Don't fret about the details. Sometimes a picture is worth a thousand words.

Carbohydrates have very simple structures that are easily broken down during digestion, which of course starts in the mouth. Carbs look like this:

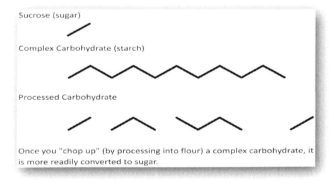

Sucrose (sugar)

Complex Carbohydrate (starch)

Processed Carbohydrate

Once you "chop up" (by processing into flour) a complex carbohydrate, it is more readily converted to sugar.

It is common knowledge that candy and soda cause cavities. Studies dating back to 1955 repeatedly show that sucrose (common table sugar) is the most virulent carbohydrate associated with cavity formation. Sucrose also changes the structure of plaque to make it stickier, so plaque can form more efficiently. However, even fructose and glucose, in high concentrations, can make cavities very quickly.

Complex carbohydrates (starches) have slipped under the dental radar for decades. A starch is more complex because it's made up of multiple glucose molecules linked together. Bacteria can still process complex carbohydrates, but it takes them longer to do so than to break down simple carbohydrates. If these complex carbohydrates stay near the teeth long enough—by frequent grazing or by being sticky enough to stay on the teeth, or both—they convert to the sugar that feeds mouth bacteria.

Sucrose causes cavities faster than starches. There is no question. Starches need more time on teeth than sugar. However, if you feed your child sticky starches multiple times a day, they will cause cavities just the same as sugar. Don't give starch the opportunity.

Processed complex carbohydrates such as flour convert very easily to sugar because the bacteria have less work to do to break it up. (Look at the diagram again.) The act of chopping up the starches with machines already did a lot of the work for the bacteria.

Refining flour takes away some of the complexity of the starch. There are fewer barriers to the sugars. But not all starchy carbs are so easy. A potato or brown rice may be capable of causing cavities but are not as likely to do so because they will be broken down much more slowly than will a food made with flour or sugar. The sugars in flour are more easily accessible to bacteria because they are already processed (chopped up) into smaller pieces.

Not all complex carbohydrates are created equal. As a rule for teeth, a whole grain of brown rice (complex carbohydrate) is better than brown rice flour (processed complex carbohydrate). Not so coincidentally, this is also true in regards to insulin. Every diabetic patient knows that crackers (which are made with flour) are a snack to spike blood sugar quickly if needed.

Fat molecules are slightly more complex and cannot cause cavities. From a biochemical standpoint, fat molecules take much too long to convert to sugar. Their molecular structure looks like this:

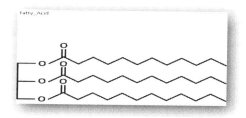

Proteins look nothing like carbohydrates. Similar to fat, protein also is not capable of causing cavities. An example of a protein molecule looks like this:

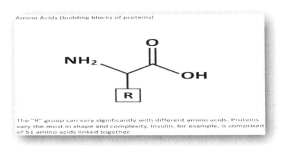

Amino Acids (building blocks of proteins)

The "R" group can vary significantly with different amino acids. Proteins vary the most in shape and complexity. Insulin, for example, is comprised of 51 amino acids linked together.

Fiber is in a category by itself. Think of fiber as an indigestible box because fiber is the plant cell wall (called cellulose) and is indigestible. If you are trying to limit bacteria's access to sugar, being trapped in a fiber cell wall is good. The box can be broken, but it is a lot of work for the both the bacteria in the mouth and in the gut to get at the food inside. This is why blood-sugar levels rise slowly when you're digesting foods with fiber. Eating fibrous foods lowers the concentration of sugar available to mouth bacteria (and fiber explains why fresh fruit is better than juice).

Faster is *not* better when it comes to sugar digestion for bacteria.

Processing whole grains into flour also processes the fiber, so the bacteria have much faster access to the carbohydrates, which are no longer hiding inside the fiber. Although whole-grain flour is better nutritionally than white flour, they are both processed carbohydrates when it comes to teeth. Whole oats are better for teeth than oat flour.

REMEMBER TIME ON TEETH

Now that you know more about how cavities form in your child's teeth (and in yours), the biggest thing to remember is that *how* you eat (grazing or organized) is as important as *what* you eat. Even fiber-rich blueberries are capable of causing cavities if you eat four blueberries every twenty minutes for eight hours every day. You shouldn't graze on fruit or any other food (such as bite-size crackers) constantly throughout the day.

Yes, crackers are convenient for toddlers to carry around, but when eaten, they turn into a mushy, starchy paste that sticks to the teeth longer than fresh fruit or fresh bread. I allow my daughter to eat crackers at preschool, but that is the only time of the day she (unlike many children) gets them. Stickiness is also why I am not worried about the cavity-causing potential of whole-grain bread or potatoes.

Technically, a potato could cause a cavity, but I don't think it will stay on the teeth long enough to do so. Most kids don't carry around bread or mashed potatoes all day long. Additionally, with bread's spongier composition, it doesn't get jammed in between the teeth as badly as crackers do. You can test this very easily. Just chew some whole-grain bread and time how long it stays on your teeth. Less than a minute. Now, chew some crackers, and time that. If you don't pick at it, it is closer to ten minutes. That's why I often make whole-grain toasted bread with peanut butter as a convenient snack. (Remember that 100 percent peanut butter with no sugar added contains close to no carbohydrates, so even though peanut butter is sticky from oil, it is not cavity causing.)

MOMS, BACTERIA, AND FOOD:

Microbiomes (the type and amount of different bacteria that live in the human body) have been getting a lot of attention recently—and for good reason (think probiotics). There are more microorganisms in your body than there are cells, and evidence suggests that the microbiome plays a bigger role in health and disease than we previously understood.

Plaque is the equivalent of a microbiome found on the teeth. I suppose you could call it a localized microbiome. Everyone has plaque. Research shows that as plaque forms, the composition of bacteria changes based on the frequency and concentration of sugars. However, even though the bacteria in the plaque play a critical role in cavity formation, we have been focusing too much on antibacterial measures.

The classic logic is: bacteria cause cavities, so we should use antibacterial mouth rinses, brush and floss more frequently to destroy the biofilm, and use more fluoride to make the teeth more resistant to acid attack from the bacteria. All of these statements are true, but doing *more* of these things doesn't fix the underlying problem.

What if the cause of so much high-risk mouth bacteria is the food we eat? What if cavity-riddled *weak teeth* are not weak at all, but the result of energized bacteria fed by the frequent consumption of easily digestible carbohydrates (such as flour and sugar)? Emerging evidence in the laboratory supports this, and my success with my patients does too.

In other words, if you change the diet, the bacteria that live on your teeth will be changed with it. In the laboratory setting, this has been shown over and over. In fact, in one study, when researchers took away all glucose, the most virulent bacteria that causes cavities (*S. mutans*) simply disappeared from the slab. In humans, we don't know how long it takes, and it's difficult to study. However, I hope more research starts from this viewpoint in the future.

DO MOMS GIVE KIDS CAVITIES?

When I was in dental school, we learned the "vertical transmission" theory of cavities. It has been shown that if the primary caretaker (usually mom) has had a recent, significant history of cavities, then the child has a much greater risk for cavities. While this correlation is well established, the specific cause is not.

The theory is that mothers pass on their bacteria to their children, giving the children a more virulent strain of bacteria, which puts them at an increased risk for cavities. To prevent this, dentists are supposed to instruct moms to not share spoons with their children. I used to advise this, too—until I had a child of my own. Then I realized that even if this vertical hypothesis were true, the recommendation was absolutely pointless. There is no possible way that a mom (or primary caretaker) is *not* going to transfer oral bacteria to her child. Is a mom never going to kiss her child on the lips? Never share a spoon? *Really*?

Also, if mom hasn't had a cavity in twenty years, shouldn't she be trying *harder* to pass on her bacteria?

The carbohydrate microbiome hypothesis—or horizontal-transmission theory—makes more sense. Mom can create a "high-caries-risk" bacterial biofilm in her mouth by frequently eating easily digestible carbohydrates. The child also creates a high-caries-risk bacterial biofilm by the same mechanism: frequently eating easily digestible carbohydrates. The correlation may exist between mother and child because mom passes on similar eating habits. Maybe the parent is not simply passing on her bacteria, but passing on her eating habits? If mom doesn't drink a lot of water, it is likely that her child won't drink a lot of water. While this is a gross oversim-plification of the research, sometimes the easiest expla-nation is the most accurate. Horizontal transmission also might explain why the ongoing fight against bacteria with traditional methods hasn't yet worked. In fact, using the latest antimicrobial varnish applied to teeth does not have a significant effect on cavity prevention.

This simplest explanation is what I've learned in my research and with the patients in my practice: **carb-rich foods** such as crackers **plus time** on teeth **equals cavities**. It's that simple. Once you know that cavity preven-tion starts in the grocery store, the implementation at home actually becomes easier. You can prevent cavities on your own by following the three simple principles outlined next in Part III.

WHY CRACKERS ARE THE LEADING CAUSE OF "SURPRISE" CAVITIES (THE CRACKER HYPOTHESIS)

I define "surprise" cavities as those not caused by candy, soda, or juice and that cause a parent to be surprised when the parent learns that their child has cavities. My clinical observation has shown that the most common cause of "surprise" cavities in children, and presumably adults, is frequent consumption of dried flour snacks such as crackers, pretzels, and dry-flour cereal. I call this the "cracker hypothesis". While not taught in dental school, the simplicity of this idea is profound. Historically, most of these surprise cavities have been blamed on weak enamel or genetics. While many good dentists have figured out that crackers are a major cavity causer, the fact that not every dentist is currently aware of it needs to change, and part of the main purpose of my writing this book is to get the message out to every dentist and parent in America. Most dentists want to help prevent cavities just as passionately as I do, and this is often the missing piece of information they need.

In fact, one of the classic dental studies from the 1950s on rats showed that sucrose (table sugar) was the most virulent cavity causer, and it used liquid starch as a control. Even the control rats in the study still had cavities; they were just not as severe and did not appear as quickly as they did in the rats given table sugar. We need to stop using the 1950s mind-set that cavities are inevitable. Liquid starch does not have to be normal food. If you think about it, dried crackers turn into liquid starch when they mix with saliva. Just as liquid starch should not be the control in a scientific experiment anymore, crackers do not have to be a staple in your child's diet anymore.

This new hypothesis easily explains most of the former surprise cavities I have encountered. I call them "surprise" cavities because dentists already know about eating candy all day, eating oranges all day, drinking soda or juice all day (or even milk all day or all night). But crackers are not even on the radar in some cases. If we simply were able to get every child to eat crackers only once a day or less, I would predict *a 50 percent cavity reduction in children under age five.*

In my own practice, the following scenario occurs at least once a week. As a pediatric dentist, I frequently get referrals from general dentists in the area when children have an excessive number of cavities or have a difficult time sitting still for a dental procedure. A dad brings in his four- or five-year-old child. His previous dentist has already informed Dad that his child has eight cavities. The dad says to me, "We brush his teeth every night. We don't give him much sugar. I am not sure where these cavities came from. I guess he just has weak teeth." I then go on to explain my hypothesis about crackers and my three prevention principles, and inevitably dad says, "Oh, that would explain it. I wish I had known that earlier."

Crackers are not inherently bad; it's just the way they are eaten that causes cavities and the fact they are extremely sticky. The problem with crackers is that they are convenient and addicting (to both parents and children). Crackers keep children occupied, kids love them, and they are presumed to be "healthy" (as opposed to sweet cookies), so kids often eat them all day long. And that brings us back, yet again, to frequency. Time on teeth is such an important variable. Oranges, for example, are just as bad for your teeth as crackers, if not worse, because of the citric acid, even though oranges are nutritious. (Dietary acids can cause cavities as well, like oranges or soda.) However, oranges usually do not create bad habits the way crackers do. It all goes back to habits. And, of course, crackers happen to be extremely sticky and stay on or in between the teeth long after they are consumed. This stickiness factor greatly adds to the amount of time that starches are touching the teeth.

What is freeing about realizing that crackers are one of the main cavity causers is that you can be less fearful of other treats such as dark chocolate and ice cream (because you won't start a bad habit of eating ice cream or chocolate all day long). There are many positives to knowing how cavities are formed. Knowledge is power, as the saying goes. I will discuss these sweets in more detail later. However, it is easy to see how many well-meaning parents shunned sugar for their children but accidentally ended up causing eight cavities anyway.

MOST SURPRISE CAVITIES HIDE IN BETWEEN TEETH

Ask any dentist who treats children if he or she has seen this pattern before: A-MO, B-DO, I-DO, J-MO, K-MO, L-DO, S-DO, T-MO. Most will say, "Every day." That is the dental shorthand for describing eight cavities hiding in between the primary molars. This pattern of cavities is one of the most common and at the same time most surprising to parents. This is the pattern that doctors' kids, dentists' kids, and nutritionists' kids can get easily. This is the exact pattern, I hypothesize, that comes from dry starches, such as crackers or cereals, getting jammed between the teeth for a few years multiple times a day. Brushing habits were probably immaculate by parents. The child could have healthy checkups for five years until this cavity pattern shows up on the first x-rays taken around ages four or five. The dentist had no reason to take x-rays earlier because everything looked immaculate on the outside of the teeth.

Sure, flossing probably would have helped. But it wasn't the lack of flossing that caused the cavities; it was the frequent starches. I have seen multiple families that flossed, but the children's frequent cracker habit was so great they still ended up with eight cavities. Cavities don't care about effort. All cavities care about are carbohydrates and time.

Change the snack foods. Change the time. Don't get surprised!

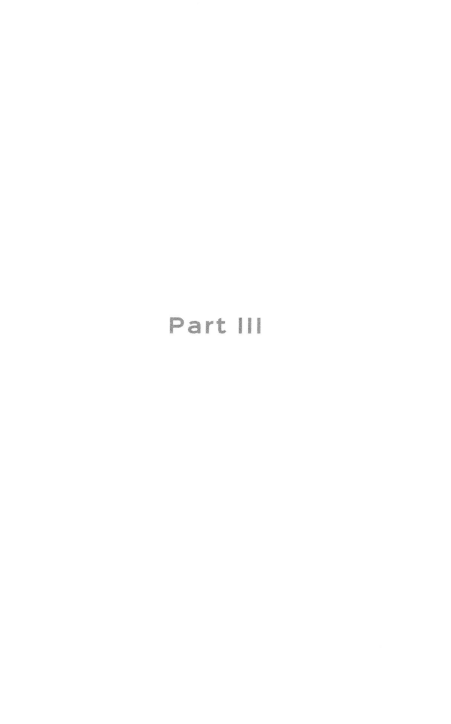

Part III

The Three Cavity-Prevention Principles

The three cavity-prevention principles I share now are based on that all-important aspect of *time*. In a simplified view, cavity prevention comes down to the twenty minutes when acid attacks teeth as part of the bacterial digestion of simple carbohydrates before saliva rinses it away. Since these principles are designed around cavity causation, if you do the opposite of them, your child will almost be guaranteed to get cavities. However, if you simply follow my three principles (plus flossing when your child's teeth begin to touch), you will surely grant your children entrance into the Cavity-Free Club.

PRINCIPLE ONE: Brush teeth every night to remove the bacteria.

Have a "perfect" brushing with help from a parent once every twenty-four hours. I suggest doing this at nighttime before bed because after this brushing, you should have nothing to eat or drink except water.

PRINCIPLE TWO: Don't graze or sip; have six "minimeals" a day and water in between.

Feed children at organized meal or snack times every few hours and have only water to drink in between meals.

PRINCIPLE THREE: Eat more dark chocolate and fewer crackers.

Know which snacks cause cavities and which snacks do not, and then snack accordingly.

I further recommend adding what I call PRINCIPLE ZERO: floss in between teeth when the teeth start touching.

That's all there is to it! You now have a simple, workable plan (but I'll explain in more detail to help make it happen).

Note: Flossing is actually not necessary for zero cavities, but it is a little added insurance. When you floss, it lets you get away with more "imperfections" in other areas. No one is perfect at everything when it comes to diet, so I still recommend flossing in areas where the teeth touch. Out of the zero-cavity kids in my practice, about half of them seem to floss and half do not, but 99 percent of them have crackers once a day or less. I honestly don't believe flossing is anywhere near as important as the quality and frequency of diet, but I don't want to experiment on my own children, and I don't recommend you experiment on yours. Floss for extra insurance when the teeth start to touch! But realize you can't outfloss a bad tooth diet.

Let's take a look at each principle in a bit more depth.

PRINCIPLE ONE: BRUSH EVERY NIGHT

Brush your child's teeth "perfectly" for twenty seconds every twenty-four hours at nighttime before bed. After this brushing, do not give your child anything to eat or drink except water. The twenty seconds that *you* brush their teeth every day until they reach the age of six or seven is more important than how often your children brush.

Why is this brushing from the parent necessary? Bacteria as a group take about twenty-four hours to grow into the sticky substance called plaque. Once plaque makes a biofilm comprised of hundreds of different types of bacteria that share nutrients synergistically, these bacteria produce lactic acid more efficiently. The more simple carbohydrates the bacteria have access to, the stickier the plaque. Brushing well once a day is the easiest way to disrupt the biofilm!

Twenty Seconds Is Enough

Brushing should serve the purpose of removing bacteria, not food. As children get older, you can work your way up to brushing two minutes twice a day, but this advice is really geared more for kids who are brushing their own teeth (ages six and up).

Sure, if you want to do the American Dental Association's recommended two minutes twice a day—go for it! Remember, however, that the snack foods you choose are more important than brushing. What about brushing after every meal? If you can, great. But with little ones, especially` if you're caring for multiple children, this is unlikely to happen. But don't worry. Changing the snack foods prevents cavities more effectively than does additional brushing.

Once you choose the right snack foods, brushing can serve its correct purpose: brushing off bacteria, not food. I spend only twenty seconds brushing my daughters' teeth every night because I am extremely selective with the snack foods they eat during the day. I choose foods that simply don't stick to the teeth. There is nothing to brush off after eating cheese and an apple. I am also very effective with my twenty seconds. I clean every surface that would get missed otherwise. For those that are wondering, all three of my daughters are still cavity-free, even though the oldest has weak enamel (hypoplasia).

My alternative view on prevention is that diet is more important than brushing. This should be everyone's view. Spend more time getting the right snacks at the grocery store, and *then* you can spend less time brushing. It only take two minutes of brushing if you give your kid crackers or other sticky foods. Test it out yourself. Just try to brush your kid's teeth immediately after they eat a cracker. It is virtually impossible. Your hand will hurt. Then, try it after they eat bread or an apple. Brushing magically turns into a lovely experience. It is absolutely a night and day difference.

Parents Should Brush Young Children's Teeth

Parents should always do the nighttime brushing. Assume that if your child is under age five, self-brushing counts as nothing. The fifteen to twenty seconds you spend is all that matters because you are still better at it. Preschoolers don't have the manual dexterity to properly reach all their teeth; they will miss the same spot over and over. However, having them brush their teeth will help form a good and necessary habit. If you want to let them brush first and then go in and do the cleanup, that is fine. Eventually, you will be ready to teach them exactly how to brush, and they will be able to take over. But don't rush it. A good rule of thumb for this transfer of power is when your child can tie his or her shoelaces. When you do decide to transfer tooth brushing responsibility to your child, make sure to check it. You wouldn't let your child drive a car without teaching him first.

For a good visual explanation of exactly how to brush, it is easier to explain in video format. Please visit TheDentistDad.com/howtobrush for a video tutorial on exactly how I hold the toothbrush and get the hard-to-reach areas in the easiest manner possible. I highly recommend that you watch this video, because you should know the ideal technique and the tricks I have learned in order to get the hard-to-reach spots in an efficient manner. Some of the ways I hold the toothbrush took me a few years to perfect, and are more effective on kids with a strong gag reflex.

Nothing Except Water After Brushing At Night

Not eating or drinking anything but water after nighttime brushing holds true for your entire life. For children, start this important habit at twelve months. I am obviously not discussing newborn babies, who must feed every few hours at night. Under age twelve months, the only hard-and-fast rule is to never leave the bottle in bed with children. Thankfully, newborns do not have teeth!

Why Nighttime Bottles Are A Problem

Saliva rinses away the acid that bacteria make. Milk, although good for your teeth, still contains lactose—a natural sugar that bacteria love. At nighttime, there is no saliva on the top teeth because of gravity. Since there is no saliva, the acid does not rinse away after twenty minutes and stays on teeth exponentially longer. When a child sleeps, one-half of the mouth is always dry because gravity causes saliva to pool on the downward side. This usually leaves the top teeth, or those on the right side or left side, dry. This is exacerbated with children who are mouth breathers because of asthma or allergies. When there is just a small amount of bacteria left on the teeth before bed, or any residual sugar (even from a small amount of milk), the acid can stay on the teeth for hours. It could be the acid equivalent of three extra snack times during the day.

Introducing sugar after nighttime brushing (even from an otherwise healthy source such as milk or formula) causes the cavity formation process to start at an early age. Ideally (if only for the teeth's sake), every child would mag-ically start sleeping through the night at twelve months or before. From my experience, a single night feeding each night between the ages of twelve and eighteen months does not seem to start early cavities but can if continued beyond eighteen months. With three or more feedings at night after twelve months, we can definitely start to see signs of cavities in some families.

Many "getting-kids-to-sleep" books say that multiple feedings of children over age eighteen months are OK. That may be just fine for the children, but unfortunately, it may not be for their teeth. And cavities at age two or three are the least fun to deal with. Please keep in mind that sleep experts don't have to deal with teeth problems.

What About Breast Milk?

Breast milk is always the best thing for your baby, hands down. Breast milk should never cause cavities. In fact, a recent long-term study showed that children who breast-fed longer had fewer cavities. But because it contains lactose, cavities could possibly still happen in *extreme* circumstances. I only see it in about 1 or 2 percent of my population. This also has been shown in a laboratory setting. I really wish it were not true, but my wishes can't change things. Out of the thousands of patients I've seen, I can count on both hands how many children (probably fewer than 1 percent of those I've seen) had cavities for which the parents or I concluded that breast milk had been a contributing factor. Thankfully, it occurs only when there is a "perfect storm" of variables colliding, which usually includes feedings more than three times a night in children over eighteen months of age. Even though no mom ever believes me until it happens, I must at least mention the issue in a cavity-prevention book, as this could account for a very small percentage of "surprise" cavities. The main variables are timing (at night), frequency, how crowded the teeth are, and frequency of other carbohydrates during the day. Breast milk is still better for the teeth than any other liquid (other than water). I don't see any difference under age one, thankfully. I have seen zero issues in my clinic with multiple breast-feedings during the day with older kids,

if moms are also following the other prevention principles very carefully. The lack of saliva at night seems to
be the x-factor.

AT WHAT AGE DO YOU START BRUSHING?

You should start brushing as soon as your child has teeth,
or at a minimum by age one. If the incisors (front four
teeth, top and bottom) are present, using a washcloth to
scrub them off at night is fine. As soon as molars (back
teeth used for chewing food) are present, it is better to
switch to a toothbrush with water. It is simply too hard to
reach the molars with anything else.

The best position to brush the teeth is with your
child on a horizontal surface, such as the changing table
(my favorite), the bed, or the floor. Stand behind the
child's head so that you can see everything really well.
If you start at age one, brushing should take only five
or ten seconds. The child may or may not enjoy it, but
you do it because you love her and don't want her to
get hurt.

Lots of kids have no problem with getting their teeth
brushed, but as a parent and as a pediatric dentist, I offer
these tips that have worked for my patients and me.

A note about fluoride toothpaste: I recommend starting fluoride toothpaste when all twenty teeth are in, usually by age three, which is later then the American Dental
Association (ADA) recommends. The risk of fluorosis (a

mild cosmetic concern in the adult teeth) is greater with fluoride ingestion under age three. The risk goes down dramatically after age three because the front permanent teeth have already calcified. However, if you do not follow my three prevention principles, such as avoiding excessive processed flour and sugar, I recommend that you follow the ADA guidelines and start fluoride toothpaste when the first teeth come in.

You may wonder why I use fluoride tooth paste at all, since my kids are avoiding crackers. The answer is: I still give my kids a lot of processed flour, just not the sticky kind. They have a lot of bread, mac and cheese, and fruit. I want the extra 20-30% help, without the side effects. That is why I stick with a rice-size smear just once every 24 hours. If you compare this with a child that uses a pea-sized amount twice a day, my child is using 75% less fluoride each day, but still getting some benefit. Based on the pain and suffering I have seen as a result from cavities, I wouldn't recommend giving up fluoride toothpaste unless you cut out all processed flour, and make sure to give your kids more vegetables than fruit. If your kids eat a paleo diet that isn't excessively fruit-heavy, that would be the ideal diet to completely cut out fluoride. I find that very few parents can make this happen long term for children.

From a practical standpoint, you may want to start fluoride toothpaste earlier for younger siblings. They get away with a little bit more, food-wise, than do the older siblings.

Under age two, use nonfluoride toothpaste if your child likes it better (and you are following the other advice in this book). If your child doesn't like it, just use water. The nonfluoride toothpaste is only a training paste. Use it only if it makes your life easier.

Alternatively, if your child is genetically more prone to cavities based on your own history, consider using fluoride toothpaste when the guidelines recommend—as soon as the teeth come in.

TWENTY-THREE TIPS TO MAKE BRUSHING MORE FUN FOR YOUR CHILD
(Don't try them all at the same time!)

1. Sing a song about brushing while you brush. Make up your own, or sing, "Brush, brush, brush your teeth. Brush them every day. Brush them up, and brush them down to keep away decay" to the tune of "Row, Row, Row Your Boat."
2. Clap when you are all done.
3. Celebrate and proclaim, "Yeah! The sugar bugs are all gone."
4. Reinforce good brushing behavior by saying, "Wonderful job opening your mouth for brushing."
5. Use two toothbrushes. Let your child choose which one she wants to hold while you use the other one.

6. Brush for less time, but have a better quality brushing. At age twelve months, it may take ten seconds to get every surface of the tooth where plaque can build.

7. Wet the toothbrush first. It softens the bristles.

8. Under age two, use nonfluoride toothpaste if your child likes it better. If your child doesn't like it, just use water. The nonfluoride toothpaste is only a training paste. Only use it if it makes your life easier.

9. Have your child watch you brush.

10. Have your child watch an older sibling brush.

11. In order to get the best view, brush your child's teeth while standing behind your child while he is lying down on a bed or changing table.

12. Try brushing your child's teeth while he is standing up.

13. Play music while brushing.

14. Give your child a choice of a different-colored toothbrush every night, even if she always makes the same choice.

15. Give your child a fist bump, high five, or big hug after every brushing.

16. Make up a brushing dance to celebrate after every brushing.

17. Use a spinning toothbrush with supervision, even if it is just for distraction while you brush with a normal toothbrush. Some kids like the vibration.

18. Start with a toothbrush when the first tooth shows up, but if you want to delay it, you can use a washcloth with purposeful scrubbing while your child has only front teeth. Switch to a toothbrush once back teeth show up.
19. Have one parent brush the teeth while another distracts the child by reading a book.
20. Keep the same routine every night (remember consistency!).
21. Make a gold-star chart. Give a star for being a "good teeth-brushing helper." Load up on garage-sale toys and use them as a reward after a certain number of gold stars.
22. Have multiple flavors of toothpaste to give your child choices.
23. If your child complains the toothpaste is "too spicy," try toothpaste that contains xylitol instead of saccharin.

If you have exhausted this list and your child is still uncooperative, you likely have what is called a strong-willed child (or your child may have a sensitive mouth). Do not fret; a strong-willed child will probably make a great leader someday. But you still have to take care of his teeth today.

UNCOOPERATIVE BRUSHERS
All of the above ideas are variations on positive reinforcement. If you have tried them all but still have a child

who is not cooperating for brushing, additional positive reinforcement can be very effective. But positive reinforcement often won't work until you know that your child is capable of having his teeth brushed without his being held down. Holding him down with a big "bear hug" for brushing is a last-case scenario and done completely out of love, but if you have tried every trick in the book, then it is a last resort for oral health. Don't feel bad if that happens to be your child's personality. Don't let other parents make you feel bad. When it comes to oral health, brushing once a day is nonnegotiable. Keep it positive and ensure your actions come from a place of love, just like when your child doesn't want his diaper changed—but you do it anyway.

When it comes to brushing toddlers' teeth, there are two types of children: uncooperative and cooperative. From my observations (and personal experience with my three daughters), it seems to have more to do with the personality of the child than parenting style. If it were all parenting style, then the same thing should work with every child, right? I can tell you from experience the same thing does not work with every child. Don't feel bad if your toddler is uncooperative about brushing.

Every child is different, and one idea may work great for one child but not for another. One method may work well for a few months, and then you may need to switch to a new one. Brushing at least once every night is important for your child's health. Just like using a car seat, brushing is not negotiable. But that doesn't mean you can't try to make it fun. As the Brad Paisley song goes, "Love starts with a toothbrush."

If a child has been cooperative at least a handful of times but then switches to become uncooperative, a gold-star chart may be a useful tool. My wife and I have found that gold-star charts are effective for habits that we want to encourage, especially for our amazing—but strong-willed—older daughter. For example, for a year my daughter was very cooperative with brushing using the gold-star chart, but then she started to run away when we tried to put on pajamas. So we switched to earning the gold star by being a good helper when getting ready for bed (which included brushing and pajamas). I realize that gold stars are not for every parent, or even for every child, but simply one possible idea. Even in my own family, gold-star charts tend to be less effective with my second daughter. We found that as a more perceptive and sensitive type, she tended to do better with more verbal and emotional positive reinforcement than with a visual chart. Use your gut, but don't give up, and keep trying different things until something works for you.

Some very well-meaning people claim your children will be traumatized if you make them brush their teeth for ten to twenty seconds while uncooperative (in a loving manner.) This is completely untrue. If I followed this logic, my daughter would never get snot wiped from her nose and would stay in same clothes for days, keep poopy diapers on, and stay up all night playing iPad. It is all about attitude. If you brush teeth as punishment, that is traumatizing. If you brush teeth out of love, it is not. A toothbrush is much gentler than a needle. Trust me.

PRINCIPLE TWO: HAVE ORGANIZED EATING; DON'T GRAZE ALL DAY

Eat five to six minimeals a day, and drink water in between those minimeals. The other way to think about this principle is *frequency, frequency, frequency*.

When I first tell parents that grazing causes cavities, most say, "Oh no, my child is a grazer." When I explain it a little more, most parents realize that their children are actually eating every two or three hours—which is what I and many dieticians recommend. It may feel like grazing to parents because they are always cleaning up and preparing things, but it is not. I define grazing as eating or drinking **anything** (other than water) more frequently than every two hours. Every twenty minutes? Grazing. Every forty minutes? Grazing. Every hour? Not as bad, but still grazing.

Now, there are many children who really do graze, and for cavity prevention, that is not a good thing. In Part II, I showed how frequency is a major factor in creating cavities because the acid produced by bacteria sticks around for about twenty minutes. Any type of carbohydrate, such as the natural sugars from milk, fresh fruits, or starchy snacks, can cause this acid attack. Grazing, otherwise known as disorganized eating, ensures that teeth stay coated in cavity-producing acid for too many hours in a day. So I'll now share age-based strategies to shift away from the grazing habit because the "grazer" has 2,433 hours in the cavity-causing "acid zone" each year, while the "organized eater" has only 608 hours. When those hours are multiplied out over the three years between ages of one and four, the grazer spends 7,300 hours in the acid zone versus 1,824 hours for the organized eater. Everyday habits are more important than those on an occasional weekend at Grandma's house. It's easy to see one of the reasons cavities are so prevalent. You could be a "perfect brusher," but with grazing, the teeth don't have a chance because the saliva cannot accommodate so much time in the acid zone. Saliva can only buffer so much acid per year. Unfortunately, the preschool-aged child happens to be the demographic most likely to graze all day long.

Common Barriers To Changing The Grazing Habit
When I tell parents no grazing, some will say, "But my nutritionist told me grazing all day is good for my metabolism." Your nutritionist meant keeping your blood sugar stable, which six small meals (or three meals and two or three snacks) accomplishes.

There are an extremely small number of foods that are OK to graze on; foods that won't cause the acid attack. Unfortunately, they are not the foods that any kid I know would graze on. For example, you can graze on broccoli or raw nuts all day, and you won't get any cavities. Broccoli will fill you up so fast that you will stop grazing, and the concentration of carbohydrates in broccoli is so low that it would not induce an acid attack anyway. Nuts contain virtually only protein and fat. But how many kids under age four are going to graze on nuts (especially since whole nuts can be a choking hazard for children) or broccoli?

You decide then to switch it to one of the best superfoods in the world: blueberries. If you graze constantly (every ten minutes) on blueberries all day long, you can get cavities from those, too. But, if you eat one hundred blueberries at breakfast, you still only get twenty minutes of acid attack on the teeth. You could also eat cheese all day and won't get a cavity, but then you would have another problem: constipation. And milk is only good for your teeth after it is in your stomach. As you can see, simply sticking with the plan of eating every two to three hours and having water in between meals is best.

What If My Child Needs To Gain Weight?

Another common concern regarding grazing comes from parents who think they have underweight children. The first question I ask is, "Is this something your doctor is concerned about or that you (the parent) are concerned about?" Most pediatricians and physicians these days are more concerned about the childhood obesity epidemic (30 percent of children in America are now obese). Most times, the physician has said, "Everything looks great. Your child is growing on the age-appropriate curve." But, when you go home, the parent side of you stares at that 10 or 20 or 30 or 40 or 49.5 percentile mark and wants to see it rise. Even though your brain heard "everything is great," you create needless worry. Usually, one can resolve this by taking out the needless worry. Ask your doctor whether you should be worried or not. If the doctor says don't worry, don't be worried.

I've noticed that the children in my practice whose parents are worried about weight tend to snack on convenient foods such as crackers or dry cereal to try to gain weight; they may also drink juice or milk throughout the day. The ironic part is that there is a good chance this strategy could sabotage the nutritional needs of the child. If your child seems small and you're worried that he or she is not gaining enough weight from the four to six nutritious meals you give him or her every day, add more good fats into the equation. Crackers, dry cereal, or most anything with flour will spike the blood sugar—it also turns to sugar on the teeth and taste buds. Most children will prefer something that is sweet over something with better nutrients, such as vegetables or fruit, or especially protein (such as chicken). Many times these children end up grazing all day on low-nutrition foods and don't eat enough nutrient-dense foods at meal times.

My recommendations: Read through all of the eating tips below for your child's particular age first (and maybe even the other ones for ideas). Additionally, I highly recommend setting up a consultation with a registered dietician for individualized useful diet tips for your situation. Realize, however, that the dietician may not be aware that some "healthy" foods still cause cavities.

Special Food And Drink Treats

It's not only what your child eats that is important; what your child drinks also matters. When I recommend only water in between meals and snacks, some parents say, "I want my children to enjoy their childhoods, so I give them hot cocoa/juice/chocolate milk whenever they want a drink." Happiness is relative. If your children grew up as Inuits in the nineteenth century and ate seal every day, they could still be really happy.

If you want to give your children something because it is a special treat, give it to them. But if you give it to them all the time, it becomes a necessity, not a special treat. Things that provide more happiness than special food or drink treats are spending quality time with children. Play games, go to the park, play dress-up. When my daughter does get a special treat such as hot chocolate after a winter walk, or candy on an airplane as we go on vacation, or even cotton candy when we are at a fair, she is very happy. It makes those occasional times special. If she got candy every day, the candy on the airplane wouldn't be so special anymore. You can have a happy, cavity-free child.

TEACH YOUR CHILDREN TO DRINK WATER WHEN THEY ARE THIRSTY

Habits are done without conscious decisions. Drinking water is a habit. Drinking juice is a habit. Once you are aware that simple juice causes more harm than good because it spikes blood sugar and contributes to cavity formation, you simply make the decision to not buy it. Your child then will get in the habit of drinking water. It really is that simple. At age twelve months (when the AAP recommends weaning from a bottle), give sippy cups with water unless it is mealtime. At meals, have one cup with water and another with whole milk (or some high fat alternative fortified with vitamin D). If you routinely put the cups back in the fridge after meals, the two cups will last all day long without any extra dish work. (If you are worried about the milk going bad, throw it away and just keep the water cup all day.) Get your child involved; have him help put the water cup in the fridge so he knows it is the routine. Some kids will protest the first few times, but once they see how putting the milk in the fridge makes you so happy, they will want to please you.

As soon as possible, switch to a normal cup.

The rule for cavity prevention is to have only water between meals. Many kids will be happy to carry the water around with them in either the bottle or sippy cup. If you make it a rule as soon as she leaves the high chair from day one, it is very, very easy to maintain because your child knows the routine.

AGE-APPROPRIATE PRACTICAL TIPS

Age One: Setting Up Good Habits

If you happen to be reading this when your child is age one or younger, that is the best time, because it is easier to *establish* healthy habits than it is to *change* unhealthy habits.

The best food habit at age one is to keep snack times organized. The second-best habit is consistency. John Medina, author of *Brain Rules for Baby*, offers this sage parenting advice: the rules you choose to apply, and even how you deal with the rules, are not as important as consistency. This is true for all aspects of parenting. So if you choose to keep snack times organized, then consistency is important to help your child learn about where and when to eat. When it comes to emotional attachment, the rules don't matter so much as long as they are consistent. When it comes to cavity prevention, the rules matter immensely. So, simply choose rules based on having healthy teeth, and stay consistent from the start.

There are many ways to have organized eating, but here's what worked best at our house. We had one area for eating: the high chair. All food was served there. If you start it now, it is very simple for the next year. Another trick at this age is to keep the snacks up high and out of sight. As soon as your child is old enough to point to the snacks that he so desperately wants but shouldn't have, you have to outsmart him (or simply not have unhealthy snacks in the house).

Eating snacks in the high chair is a great habit to begin. If you never have food anywhere else, there is no fuss. By eighteen months, toddlers are walking around. If unknowing parents keep crackers and cereals in the pantry, the child will see them and want them. When you say no, a tantrum may result. Since she's too young for time-outs, and she doesn't understand the logic of your explanation that she can't have crackers, she will continue to point at that delectable box of crackers (or cereal) with a quivering lip and a high-pitched squeal. When this day inevitably occurs, that is when it is important to remember how destructive grazing can be to the teeth. That is the day when unknowing parents start that destructive habit because they don't even know it is bad. You, however, do know, so you can make a good choice for your child's teeth.

If it's time for snack, go ahead and put her in the high chair (or predetermined snack area) and have a snack. If it's not snack or mealtime, you will have to consistently say no. The easiest trick is "out of sight, out of mind." Simply move snacks somewhere where they won't be seen. You should now be good until age two, when she gets so smart she realizes it's hidden in the top cupboard or knows how to ask for it. If cavities are an unacceptable outcome for you, it's best to not have crackers in the house and stock only foods you want her to eat. This pithy statement sounds completely outside the norm because it is. Remember the statistics: over 60 percent of five-year-olds in America have a cavity. You have to be a little different from "normal" to keep your kids cavity-free, and the *easiest*, most *practical* step is to keep crackers out of the house. Every parent has a limit on how many times she wants to say no each day, so it is better to set yourself up for success.

Formula And Milk In Nighttime Feedings

Formula and milk have definitely been shown to contribute to cavities. When parents share that their twelve-month-old child is feeding four times or more a night, I will explain the cavity process, make sure everything else is in order, and recommend trying to wean the child from the nighttime feedings before eighteen months. If it is still happening at eighteen months, then

I offer stronger encouragement to stop the nighttime feedings for those using formula or cow's milk. This is partly because I often see cavities forming early on when children are feeding multiple times at night.

Thankfully, for children younger than a year old, nighttime feeding doesn't make any difference for teeth as long as you don't leave the bottle in the bed. If the bottle is left in the bed, usually by the time I see the child, it is too late to save the teeth. Instead, it requires general anesthesia to fix them or simply relieve the child from pain. Never leave the bottle in bed with your child.

One final note: even if an eighteen-month-old's multiple feedings don't cause cavities, it could weaken the child's enamel, thus starting the cavity process early. The teeth could be more prone to cavities over the next three years and would need more intervention than would teeth that did not have two to three hours of acid attacks every night for months. Starting in-office fluoride varnishes earlier (at age one) could be beneficial for children at high risk for cavities. If you are on the edge of deciding when to transition into a longer nighttime sleeping pattern, the teeth would prefer sooner rather than later.

Age Two: The Importance Of Water

If your child does not learn how to drink water when he is thirsty, you might as well plan on cavities. Imagine two children. One child has a sip of water after every snack or meal, essentially cutting down the twenty-minute acid attack from the food to five minutes. The second child has a sip of watered-down juice after every meal, prolonging the twenty-minute acid attack. Not only that, the second child has a sip of watered-down juice a few times between meals, adding additional twenty-minute acid attacks. Which child is going to have "weak enamel"? The child who gave his or her teeth very mild yet frequent acid attacks, of course.

Don't water down juice. Diluting juice gives a false sense of security. I learned this the hard way when I used to recommend this to parents. If you start to water down juice, your child will think it is water, and it will be very difficult to go back to just water. Watering down juice ends up backfiring and creating more cavities instead of fewer. Don't let her get confused. If she is sick with a cold, just provide her with 100 percent juice for two straight days to avoid dehydration if needed, and then switch back to water when she is better. I give my children juice in their beds when they are sick with a fever, but this practice obviously goes back to normal when health returns.

The easiest way to develop a water habit is to remove all temptation of other options. Simply don't have the apple or orange juice in the house until you know you can limit it to meal times. Even then, having juice three meals a day is too much liquid sugar for the teeth.

Although I am anti-juice for the sake of preventing cavities, I am pro-smoothies. The reason is mostly psychological and partly nutritional. I still recommend limiting them to once a day, maybe twice at most. Technically, a smoothie is just fancier, more expensive juice. However, since the smoothie is so amazingly delicious, kids often will gulp down the whole thing (meaning only a few seconds on the teeth). Kids might ask for smoothies at every meal or snack time the way they will ask for juice, but for parents, it is easier to say no to an expensive smoothie—especially a handmade smoothie—when compared with apple juice, which is almost as cheap as water. Cost (and work) limits the supply of smoothies. Because apple juice is so easy and inexpensive, it is emotionally more difficult for parents to say no when compared with a request for a smoothie. The other added benefit of a smoothie is that it is thicker than water, so it is not easily confused with water. Kids should always associate having water with quenching their thirst. Regular juice blurs the thirst-quenching line too easily. Smoothies are OK because it is easy to limit them to five minutes a day.

My wife is quite amazing. And she's very good at making smoothies from scratch, too. She takes a bunch of berries, a little yogurt, even some spinach, and a little flaxseed oil for good fat (which can be good for the brain and digestion, too) for a dynamite smoothie. Since I am an ordinary human being and too lazy to make a smoothie from scratch, I buy smoothies at the grocery store. This seems expensive at first, but I end up giving much less volume to my daughters than I do when serving regular juice. Cavities can be expensive financially and emotionally, so if you count the dental bill as well, I end up saving money and cavities. We fortify our smoothies by adding flaxseed oil to gain good omega-3 fatty acids.

My main nutritional criterion for smoothies is to have fiber in it. Smoothies contain more fiber because they contain the whole fruit, not just the juice. (Not all store-bought smoothies have fiber—check the label before you buy it.) The fiber helps lessen the spike in blood sugar, helps fill you up the natural way, and helps prevent constipation. Constipation, by the way, is the number one cause for emergency room visits in children. I learned this after spending two days on an emergency room rotation for my pediatric residency. Ask any emergency room nurse or doctor. Most kids don't get enough fiber.

Remember, consistency is the key to developing good habits. Stick with only water between minimeals. Once you establish the rule, it will be easier to maintain. I also would still try to limit smoothies to once a day, or twice at most.

Age Three: Good Habits Continue

Continue to brush your child's teeth. Your child brushing his own teeth is not a developmental milestone. At least, if you want to prevent cavities, you won't pass that baton on this early. At ages three and four, and even five and six, children still need parental assistance to brush properly. It is good for them to want to do it themselves, but after they are done with their turn, you must get in there and get the many spots they missed. The ten to twenty seconds of brushing that you do every night is more important than your child's brushing his own teeth a few times a day. When your child is old enough to brush on their own, after age six, have them transition to the two-minute brushings twice a day. Since I am a diet-focused dentist and dad, we don't make it the full four minutes in a day, but I still help out my six-year-old at night to make up for it. My philosophy is that it is more important to have one "perfect" cleaning once every twenty-four hours, and the amount of time it takes you isn't the most important factor. (This is based on that plaque takes about 24 hours to form). I let my daughter brush her teeth on her own in the morning.

By age three there is often some visible or invisible damage that has already been done if your child has been sipping on milk, juice, or watered-down juice throughout the day for the past two years. Depending on the frequency, cavities may be present, but they're invisible without an x-ray. You are not the first parent to fall into this category, nor will you be the last. Either way, it is good to start the prevention principles right now, in order to still have a chance to prevent further cavities or to delay the need to fix the forming cavities. It is much easier to fix cavities in five-year-olds than in three- or even four-year-olds.

If you have already started the habit of water between meals, continue it. If your child has had anything else between meals, switch to water straightaway. Nothing causes cavities faster than drinking liquid forms of sugar frequently, even if they are natural.

Ages Four, Five, And Up

If you started earlier, by age four you have already instilled good habits. Your child knows that brushing teeth is not a negotiable item. You have established specific organized snack times, and you give your kids teeth-friendly foods. Because good habits have already been set, you can go into maintenance mode.

But what if you, like millions of other parents, did not start thinking about cavities until they already happened, and you want to change into healthy-teeth habits now? You can't prevent the cavities that have already started forming, but you can prevent cavities in the adult molars that come in at age six. You also may be able to greatly decrease the rate of growth of any cavities that have already started. It is possible to stop cavities from growing with extra fluoride and an extremely low-carb diet.

It is just extremely difficult to do so because the layer underneath enamel is much weaker than enamel itself.

First, make sure you and your spouse are on the same page. Cooperative parenting always strengthens your position when change is necessary. Then focus on the foods you buy at the grocery store, and focus on implementing the three prevention principles. If there is a day care, nanny, or other caretaker involved, keep them in the loop. Print out my snack guide at TheDentistDad. com/snackguide and give it to them. Give them a copy of this book.

Second, explain to your children that your doctor (or this book) has taught you the difference between snacks that are healthy for teeth and snacks that are not. Since you want your children to have healthy teeth, you're changing the snack rules so they won't get any (more) cavities.

As you make changes, it's important that you do not label foods as good or bad. There are no bad foods. There are just some foods we have all the time and some foods we have some of the time. You don't want to encourage feelings of guilt about food at an early age. Crackers are not horrible for you; they just cause cavities if you eat them too frequently. Milk is good for your teeth at mealtimes, but if you are thirsty at other times, you should drink water. Bacon is great for your teeth because it is mostly fat, but you don't want to eat that all day long either. I often tell my children, "It's good to eat a variety of foods each day."

Focus on the fun stuff you will still do. For example, you can say, "We will no longer eat crackers all day, but we can have a piece of dark chocolate some days after lunch instead." (Cutting down from five starch episodes to one sugar/fat episode is actually a large improvement.) Or, "We won't eat potato chips all afternoon, but we can go out for ice cream on Fridays." In other words, you will be taking away some things they like, but you will be adding other fun things to replace them. When you compromise and give your child sweets, be strategic about it and choose ice cream or dark chocolate. (I will discuss these treats in more detail later.) This is how you work the system: make sure the sugar is not on the teeth for long, in order to "get away" with it. Most types of candy are still bad for teeth, of course, because they are sticky or last a long time.

Of course, if you can switch your dessert to fresh raspberries, that would be ideal, nutritionally. I just haven't done that yet.

If you are in the minority and your children have made it to age five without cavities, congratulations! Most children who make it to five with zero cavities can easily stay cavity-free to age ten and beyond. This is because the healthy habits just keep going. You are drinking water as a habit. You are eating healthy snacks and brushing every night. Additionally, once children are school age, they can't graze on crackers all day. And if your child is one of those more sensitive, anxious, or "gaggy" kids, you have lots of motivation to keep your zero-cavity streak perfect (in order to avoid time in the chair having dental work done), so keep those good habits going strong.

AVOIDING THE YOUNGER-SIBLING-CAVITIES TREND

Most of the time, younger siblings get more cavities than do older siblings. I cannot tell you how many times I have had families in which the oldest child (or children) had zero cavities at age eight. Then, like clockwork, the youngest sibling turns five and is finally able to have x-rays to check for cavities hiding in between the teeth, and I find eight cavities. The cavities usually present in pairs of two and are in all four likely spots. Then the mother or father, looking shocked, says, "But I did everything the same!" I used to shrug and say, "It's weak enamel." That was before I discovered the "cracker hypothesis." Once you change your paradigm, the answer becomes obvious.

How can you avoid this sibling trend? Here is my extremely scientific reasoning about why younger siblings get more cavities than do older siblings: we give younger siblings crackers to keep them quiet.

Doesn't that make sense? Firstborn children are often fed fresh fruits and vegetables (from your organic garden in the backyard, of course). By the third kid, you hardly have time for food shopping, let alone taking a shower, so you push a bowl of crackers in front of the little one to keep him quiet as you rush to fill everyone's needs. It's not an indictment, just a reality. I joke with parents, telling them to give younger siblings tablets to keep them quiet; they might get ADHD, but at least they won't have holes in their teeth. My joke is sarcastic but partially true in my own household. Setting limits on screen time is important, too. Letting kids learn how to entertain themselves without food or electronics is an important life skill.

There are a few other reasons for the younger-sibling trend:

Younger siblings start most things at a younger age. Take juice, for example. If you were super awesome and waited until age five to serve apple juice (other than special occasions or bouts of sickness), you deserve the biggest parental pat on the back ever because absolutely none of your friends did such a thing. But the youngest sibling somehow starts getting juice at age two. This is simply one example, but my point is obvious: it is emotionally and practically more difficult to do things "exactly" the same as you did with your firstborn.

The biggest reason that younger sibling get more cavities, however, is the lack of awareness of the cracker hypothesis. You attribute your older children's zero-cavities success to a relative dearth of candy, absolutely no soda, virtually no juice, and strong enamel. You don't remember that your older children did not graze on crackers all day.

"But I got away with not flossing with my other kids," you say. And, in fact, you did. So you knew you would be set with the second (or third) child because your children have genetically superior teeth. But combine no flossing with extra crackers and more juice, and you have the perfect setup for eight cavities at age five for the youngest sibling. Another way of stating the theory is that you got away with not flossing your first child's teeth *because* she didn't have crackers very often, didn't graze often, and had more water. Since your first child, you've made other subtle changes, and, all of sudden, you could not get away with not flossing (imagine flour jammed in between the teeth for two years).

So if you want to be proactive and keep up your zero-cavity streak for your youngest children (which would be impressive with two children, amazing in three children, and otherworldly with four or more), I would focus on the three principles starting at age one. Keep the "snacking only in certain places and times" habit going. Keep the rule of only carrying around water (not even milk is allowed away from the table). And because, by default, you are going to be more imperfect with the younger children, perhaps even floss their teeth even though you did not floss the older kids' teeth.

I am happy to report that since I have been informing parents about my prevention principles for the past few years, I have had hundreds of families make it successfully to even the third (or fourth) child with zero cavities by age five. My theories have been working in my practice, and I have fewer surprised parents. Even more importantly, I have helped countless families completely reverse the trend. Their eldest child had eight cavities, and they were able to keep the youngest child cavity-free by changing all of the unhealthy habits. In most cases, bad genetics can be overcome with enough effort started early.

HOW TO STOP "JUICING" YOUR KID IF YOU'VE ALREADY STARTED

Since juice is such a cavity culprit for young children, it's important to wean your child from reliance on juice as a staple in his or her diet.

Step one (optional): enlist outside authorities. Go to the dentist and ask her or him to specifically say, "You need to drink water between meals." Another option is a free *Sesame Street* episode called "Healthy Teeth, Healthy Me," which you can watch with your child. It talks about the importance of good oral health (go to TheDentistDad.com/resources for the link). The idea is to find some outside authorities to help prime your child for what is about to happen. Sometimes it just helps hearing from someone other than Mom.

Step two (required): explain to your child that, starting today, your family has new rules regarding juice. It is only allowed at mealtimes (hopefully, no more than once a day). In between meals, water is the only drink she can carry around. Explain that water is very good for teeth, and juice is not good for teeth. Feel free to put all of the "blame" on the dentist. Explain that you know it is frustrating, but the dentist said that juice causes sugar bugs too quickly, so you are going to have water between meals and maybe even a special smoothie at breakfast instead of juice (if you haven't already started, now may be a good time to start the habit of a sip of water after every meal as well).

What most likely will happen is that your child will stare blankly at you or maybe say OK. But that very first time you refuse to give juice, a tantrum may (or may not) ensue. Then, you get to decide which parenting strategy works best for you: distraction, ignoring, explaining again, a time-out, or a time-in. Whatever you do, stay strong. The initial frustration you may experience when trying to change habits is worth it in order to not get holes in your child's teeth.

On a public health note, juice is still considered a serving of fruit, but it is not nutritionally equivalent to fruit. And it can wreak havoc on children's teeth. While well-intentioned programs give out apple juice to mothers with low incomes because it is more practical than distributing fresh apples, it is shortsighted and simply wrong. It's a case of a program that is trying to be helpful but ends up being harmful when children get more cavities. Toddlers who live in low-income households are more likely to carry around juice than water in a sipping container even before participating in programs that make it readily available. Children in low-income households are already more prone to cavities for a variety of reasons (both parents working, fresh foods being harder to get than packaged foods). Let's not continue to compound the problem by giving them cavity-causing juice that they should not be drinking anyway.

Now, let's not discredit the other wonderful things that community programs do for young parents in need. It is not the community programs' fault they are handing out apple juice to kids and contributing to painful teeth issues. They didn't know, and they are providing food and beverages based on nutritional guidelines, not on dental health. But simply giving out applesauce instead of apple juice could make a massive public health difference. Applesauce is similar to a premade apple smoothie. And applesauce is eaten out of a bowl or packet, so it doesn't get confused with juice. The apple farmers can still be happy, and we aren't handing out cavities to low-income children. If we get enough dentists, nutritionists, and doctors onboard, hopefully we can make this change together. If juice is being handed out for free as part of any food program across the country, it needs to stop for the sake of low-income children. If you have any influence with nutritional programs, consider making a simple change from juice to applesauce for the sake of children's oral health.

The same is true for crackers. Switching to whole loaves of bread instead of boxes of crackers would be giving out easy nutrition, but with less painful consequences.

Review of Principle 2

Eat only at meal or snack times, and have water between meals. Eat every two to three hours, not every twenty minutes, because the amount of time food spends on your children's teeth matters (frequency, frequency, frequency).

PRINCIPLE THREE: EAT TEETH-FRIENDLY FOODS

Eat more chocolate, fewer crackers.

The most important aspect of this third principle is that if you want to prevent cavities and have fewer *sneaky* cavity causers in your kids' diet, the kinds of foods you eat matter. In this section, I provide a list of foods to eat less of (because they cause cavities) and a list of foods to eat more of (because they don't). In the middle, are foods that usually won't cause cavities. At the end of the day, anything with carbohydrates has the inherent ability to cause cavities, but some foods make it easier than others.

Saying that diet can prevent cavities is currently a controversial statement in dentistry. However, you will see that it should not be controversial at all. It is simply a paradigm shift. Every dentist knows that foods such as cheese neutralize the acids that cavity-causing foods make. These same dentists, because of the nutritional stigma against fat for the past half century, have just not made the paradigm shift to recognize that other low-carbohydrate foods also prevent cavities.

The good news is that we really only have to talk about snack foods. You don't have to completely over-haul your family's diet if you know how to work the sys-tem. Typically, cavities are not caused by foods we eat at mealtimes. For example, chicken and broccoli are not going to cause cavities because they are very low in carbohydrate concentration. Of course, if you are hav-ing snack foods with each meal, then you may want to consider changing those. But let's just focus on snack time because that is generally where most cavities come from. Hopefully, at this point, it is apparent how impor-tant it is to stick with the essence of principle two: keep snacks at snack times. But you will add greatly to your success when you choose the right snack foods. Before we delve into discussing different foods, let's bring up the elephant in the room, nutrition.

Nutrition And Cavity Prevention Don't Have To Match

We will soon talk about specific foods, but before we do, let's admit one thing so you, I, and other health-care professionals can have a frank discussion about cavity prevention. Nutrition and cavity prevention don't always go together, and that is OK. Ideally, they do, since the goal is to have more whole foods and fewer processed foods. We can all agree on that. However, nutrition-ists may compromise by recommending foods that are nutritious but not great for teeth. I will compromise on a few foods that are not nutritious but aren't as bad for teeth as an orange is, for example. Practicing modera-tion and variety is key. We have to admit the fact that something like an orange offers nutritional value but is not good for your teeth. On the flip side, if teeth can handle the occasional orange, then teeth can handle occasional man-made sugars, even if not nutritious. You have to be just as careful with the orange as you do with man-made sugar. The other major consideration is how sticky foods are, which is why bread is better than crack-ers even though they are almost equivalent nutritionally.

How much processing is done is also important. Whole oats are better than oat flour. Raw kale is better than kale juice. If your long-term plan is to prevent cavities, you need to think about how food affects teeth.

Different Categories Of Food For Teeth

For the purpose of causing cavities, foods fit into four different categories:

1. Foods that never cause cavities
2. Foods that won't cause cavities but are technically capable of doing so
3. Healthy foods that can cause cavities very quickly
4. Foods that cause cavities very quickly

Beverages also fit into four categories:

1. Beverages that never cause cavities
2. Beverages that can cause cavities very quickly but won't
3. Beverages that can cause cavities very quickly and will
4. Beverages that can cause cavities very slowly

For a printable version of my snack guide, visit TheDentistDad.com/snackguide.

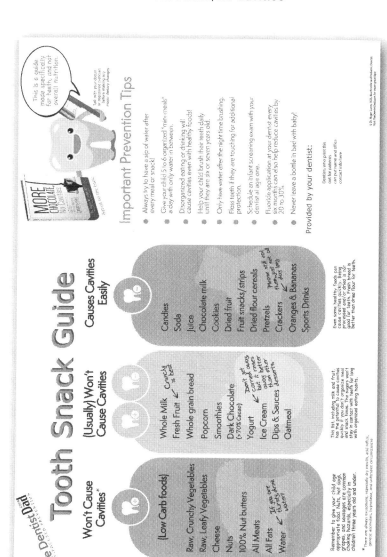

The Dentist Dad

Tooth Snack Guide

Won't Cause Cavities*

[Low Carb foods]

Raw, Crunchy Vegetables

Raw, Leafy Vegetables

Cheese

Nuts

100% Nut butters

All Meats

All Fats — *If you are thirsty drink water*

Water

Remember to give your child age appropriate food. Nuts, hot dogs, grapes, and sausages are common choking hazards, especially in children three years old and under.

*There are always exceptions, especially dry mouth, acid reflux, generic anomalies, hypoplasia, and unforeseen circumstances.

(Usually) Won't Cause Cavities

Whole Milk — *Crunchy is best*

Fresh Fruit

Whole grain bread

Popcorn

Smoothies

Dark Chocolate (>70% Cacao)

Yogurt — *Don't get cavities away but it's better away than other desserts.*

Ice Cream

Dips & Sauces

Oatmeal

This list, including milk and fruit, has the potential to cause cavities quickly if you don't organize meal and snack times. The sugars won't stay in contact with teeth for long with organized eating habits.

Causes Cavities Easily

Candies

Soda

Juice

Chocolate milk

Cookies

Dried fruit

Fruit snacks/strips

Dried flour cereals

Pretzels — *these will not sit in your mouth long*

Crackers

Oranges & Bananas

Sports Drinks

Even some healthy foods can cause cavities quickly. Being processed and/or dried is not good for teeth. Fresh bread is better than dried flour for teeth.

This is a guide made specifically for teeth, and not overall nutrition.

Talk with your doctor or registered nutritionist before making any major dietary changes.

Important Prevention Tips

- Always try to have a sip of water after every meal or snack!

- Give your child 5 to 6 organized "non-sneaky" a day with only water in between.

- Disorganized eating or drinking will cause cavities, even with healthy foods!

- Help your child brush their teeth daily until they are six or seven years old.

- Only have water after the night time brushing.

- Floss teeth if they are touching for additional protection.

- Schedule an infant screening exam with your dentist at age one.

- Fluoride application at your dentist every six months can also help reduce cavities by 20 to 30%.

- Never leave a bottle in bed with baby!

Provided by your dentist:

Dentists who print this out for patients can put name and office contact info here

© Dr. Roger Lucas, DDS, Board-certified Pediatric Dentist. Visit TheDentistDad.com for more great tips!

Cavity-Causing Foods And Beverages List

Can't Cause Cavities	Difficult to Cause Cavities but Theoretically Capable[2]	Easy to Cause Cavities
Water, unsweetened tea	Whole milk	Juice, soda, Gatorade, sweetened tea, sweetened waters, chocolate milk.
Nuts and seeds, 100 percent nut butters	Nut butters with honey or sugar	
Raw Green leafy vegetables, broccoli, carrots, and crunchy vegetables like celery.	Apples, pears, blueberries, blackberries, raspberries	Oranges, bananas, dried fruits, freeze-dried fruits
Cheese	Cottage cheese, yogurt, frozen yogurt, ice cream	Smoothies,[3] juices
100 percent cocoa with no sugar added	70 percent dark chocolate, milk chocolate, peanut-butter-based candies	Suckers, lollipops, cotton candy, sour candies, hard candies, chewy candies, fruit snacks
	Shredded wheat, rolled oats	Any type of dry-flour crackers or cereals
	Whole-grain bread	Crackers, white bread
	Dipping sauces for vegetables	
All Meats	Sauces (BBQ, Teriyaki)	
All Fats		

*Although artificial sweeteners won't cause cavities, they may make your child crave more sweet liquids. I recommend avoiding artificial sweeteners, as humans were designed to drink water.

---

2 The main idea of the middle category is that you still don't want to have this group all day long. Yogurt from the store with added sugar would definitely cause cavities if it was on your teeth all day or all night, but because of the way it is eaten, it won't be. Milk is actually a very common cause of cavities because preschoolers will carry milk around all day or have it all night. This list assumes you are keeping snack time organized.

3 Smoothies technically can cause cavities very quickly, but, in practice, they won't because they are too difficult to carry around all day (unlike plain juice), and smoothies are not confused with water.

1. Whole Foods That Never Cause Cavities

Foods that never cause cavities either contain exclusively protein and fat or have such a low carbohydrate concentration that the acidic concentration won't get high enough to cause cavities.

It's the relative *concentration* of carbohydrates that is important. As an illustration, imagine a glass of water. If you drop a slice of lemon in the water, you will have a very low concentration of carbohydrates in the water. Is this enough to lower the pH of your enamel significantly? No. What if you squeeze the lemon a little? Still, there is enough water to dilute the concentration of carbohydrates significantly enough to keep the water from damaging your teeth. If you keep pouring lemon juice into the glass, eventually you will reach a tipping point that shifts the balance into an unhealthy range for your teeth.

Here is the really interesting thing. Adding enough fat is the equivalent of lowering the simple carbohydrate concentration. A recent study compared whole, 2 percent, and skim milk given to bacteria sitting on cut-out teeth. In the lab setting, the bacteria exposed to whole milk did not produce enough acid to weaken enamel, but the bacteria in 2 percent and skim milk did. The extra fat in whole milk lowered the ratio of simple carbohydrates that the bacteria had to process, and they were too busy processing the fat to make enough lactic acid. When it comes to teeth, the more fat, the better! (Whole milk still contains some sugar, so keep it at mealtimes nonetheless.)

Whole foods are generally healthy. But if you turned kale into juice and sipped on it all day, you could find a way to make cavities because the small amount of carbohydrates contained in the kale have been released from the walls of the fiber, and sipping the smoothie all day would keep the carbohydrates on your teeth. So don't do that! Just have the kale smoothie at breakfast or eat the kale raw.

Foods that won't cause cavities include:

Nuts and seeds, green leafy vegetables, crunchy vegetables, and cheese

Nuts and seeds: Nuts and seeds are basically comprised of just protein and fat. (They have a very low carbohydrate concentration.) Since there are effectively no carbohydrates to make lactic acid, the bacteria can never produce enough acid to weaken teeth's enamel. The good news is that peanut butter and other nut butters fit into this category as well. Peanut butter is sticky from oil (not from starch), so even if it gets stuck in between your teeth, it can't cause cavities (assuming it is a peanut butter without any added sugar). Most commercial peanut butters add sugar or honey. Technically, this could cause cavities. However, I would argue that peanut butter with a little sugar added is still better than most other snacks because the concentration of sugar is relatively low when compared with fat. Still, nut butters without added sugar are better. To be safe, buy peanut butter without added sweeteners. If you want it to be easier to spread, try varieties that add coconut oil to make it more spreadable (by lessening the separation of the oils). Another trick is to store the peanut butter jar upside down. This moves all the oil to the "bottom" of the jar. Many fights in marriages revolve around which type of peanut butter to buy. If it makes you feel better, I buy the natural stuff for me, but I don't throw out the peanut butter with a little sugar added when my wife buys it.

Green, leafy vegetables and crunchy vegetables: Although some carbohydrates are present in these foods, it is a minimal amount. The fiber and water lower the *concentration* of carbohydrates dramatically enough so that there isn't enough sugar for the bacteria to process. Additionally, the fiber makes these foods self-limiting. After a certain point, you can't eat any more broccoli because your stomach is distended. Between the low-carbohydrate concentration and the inability to eat it for long periods of time, your teeth will be safe from acid attack. Elmo, from *Sesame Street*, says it best: "With crunchy fruits and vegetables, you can't go wrong."

Cheese: Cheese is virtually all protein and fat. No carbohydrates, so no acid attack. If you eat cheese all day, you will get constipated (so don't do that), but you won't get cavities.

Tip: Eat cheese after fruit for extra credit. The cheese helps balance the pH, because bacteria will start processing fat instead of sugars.

2. Foods That Won't Cause Cavities (But Technically Can)

These foods are on the "won't cause cavities" list, but technically, they contain enough carbohydrates to cause cavities if left on the teeth:

- Crunchy fruits (apples and pears)
- Noncrunchy fruits (berries) other than bananas, oranges
- Starchy vegetables (potatoes)
- Whole-grain bread
- Pasta

Apples are a good example. They technically have enough sugar to cause cavities, but they won't if you eat an apple once or twice a day, have a sip of water afterward, and follow the other principles. The fiber scrapes your teeth. The fiber also fills you up, so you won't eat apples all day long. If you found a way to eat apples five or six times a day, it would be possible to get a cavity. But if you spend five minutes eating an apple twice a day, that is only two twenty-minute acid attacks. It is even better if you complement the fruit with fats, such as cheese or peanut butter. Cheese and fruit sounds like a good combination, doesn't it?

Try to stick with the idea to incorporate a rainbow of fruits and vegetables into your kid's diet. Having a variety of colors is a good rule of thumb.

Fibrous, noncrunchy fresh fruits such as blueberries, blackberries, raspberries, apricots, plums, and most other fruits you can think of also fall into this category. With these fruits, as with all carbohydrates, it's all about frequency. If you eat one hundred blueberries for breakfast, it only counts as one acid attack. If you were to give your child a ziplock bag of blueberries to carry around and she ate one every five minutes for eight hours for 365 days, her teeth would fall apart. However, you would likely have to force feed your child to do this. So let her do her own eating during snack time and have a sip of water afterward, and you will be fine.

As far as teeth are concerned, potatoes, rice, whole-grain bread, and pasta all fit into the same basic category. They can cause cavities if you eat them all day. For example, if you lived and worked on a rice farm, it would be difficult to stay cavity-free because of the frequent rice eating. However, based on my observations, these kinds of foods are usually not a concern when eaten during mealtimes. Of course, this is assuming the meals are balanced. For example, if you lived on a rice farm and ate only rice, this would not be a balanced diet. The cavities may take years instead of months to develop, but eating rice throughout the day is a slow, gradual way to form cavities.

In a like manner, if you only ate bread, pancakes, muffins, pasta, and potatoes, your diet would not be very balanced, and the chance for cavities would increase (though they again would develop more slowly when compared with the consumption of liquid, or "stickier," carbohydrates). Baked potatoes and rice are (generally) unprocessed, so the starches are less broken down when compared with those in whole-grain bread and pasta, which are made from processed flour (which is typically not a good thing for teeth). Despite all of this, you should not be overly worried about these foods causing cavities for children because they are eaten only at mealtimes and don't stay on the teeth long (in contrast to dry crackers, which do stick to teeth). Usually breads, pastas, and rice should only cause three twenty-minute acid episodes at most. I would not worry about macaroni and cheese, spaghetti, or whole-grain bread when it comes to teeth, thankfully. And the typical American meal generally includes meat and vegetables along with the starches. Vegetarians can replace meats with other proteins and fats.

Breakfast seems to be the meal that could include the "stickiest" carbohydrates, such as syrup or cereal made from dry flour. I would recommend not having a dry flour cereal every morning. Can you get away with a dry flour cereal every morning and still get zero cavities? Of course you can, but it is just one more variable in favor of cavities. In my family, my daughter already gets crackers at preschool every day. I don't want to "double" the daily cavity-causing foods for her for the first five years of her life, when children are most prone to cavities, especially since genetics are stacked against her—both my wife and I had multiple cavities growing up. For cereals I recommend shredded wheat or oatmeal that has no added sugar (flavor with applesauce and cinnamon, and kids won't miss the sugar). If you want to know what we buy, it's a shredded-wheat cereal that has a sprinkling of powdered sugar on it, or oatmeal with some brown sugar. I'm more worried about cereal made from 100 percent dry flour than a sprinkling of sugar on top of shredded wheat or brown sugar on oatmeal because they don't stick between the teeth the way dry flour does. Full confession: We did oatmeal with applesauce for our first daughter and have "regressed" to brown sugar after having a third.

However, focusing on breakfast is for extra credit. I do not focus on it when speaking with my patients because snacks usually comprise three eating episodes a day versus breakfast's single attack. Also, not all of my patients are gung ho about achieving zero cavities for their children. I still want to help them achieve zero cavities even if the parents are not that interested. Hence, focusing on cavity-preventing snack foods is three times as effective. Yet every little thing can make a difference over a three-year period. And since the easiest time to start a good breakfast habit is as soon as possible, if you never introduce a particular type of dry cereal, your kids won't even know it's an option until they are older. Or, alternatively, use the cereal as a finger food under age one, as most parents do, but switch to a different one when you start giving them a bowl and spoon.

Yogurt

If you buy "traditional" yogurt with fruit on the bottom, the sugar content is fairly high. That is the bad news. The good news is that the sugar should rinse off the teeth quickly and yogurt is usually eaten within a five-minute period. So when it comes to teeth, similarly to fresh fruit, I wouldn't worry too much about yogurt. Eat it in five minutes, drink some water afterward, and the acid attack is done. If you are going for extra credit, buy plain yogurt and add fresh fruit yourself.

Bananas, oranges, and other citrus fruits

Bananas and oranges are good for you but have the potential to cause cavities quickly if eaten multiple times a day. Bananas are very sticky and relatively high in sugar. Oranges are very acidic, and citric acid can weaken your enamel even without sugar. Every dentist has had a few patients who have been surprised with several cavities that resulted from snacking on oranges throughout the day.

Since (as you know by now) cavity formation comes down to frequency of food or drinks touching the teeth, two oranges at breakfast should be no big deal if your child has a sip of water afterward. In fact, the vitamin C is good for the health of gums. But if you give bananas or oranges for three snacks a day, that could be a problem. And if your child sucked on oranges all day long, his teeth would fall apart in a matter of months, regardless of his brushing habits. To be on the safe side, I would rather have oranges only every other day instead of every day if I am looking at a two-year period of time.

Other Foods That Cause Cavities Very Quickly

- Most candies
- Crackers

- Dried fruit
- Processed dried fruit snacks

Most candies are high in sugar and not much else. These are the obvious cavity causers. Hard candies and suckers are probably the worst because they take a long time to dissolve. Sticky candies are right up there because they stick.

Not all candies are created equal. Milk chocolate, for example, has a higher fat content than hard candies. And there is a higher concentration of sugar in a dried fruit snack because, once you take all the water out of the fruit, the concentration of the sugar increases. You may think that a dried fruit snack is better for your teeth than chocolate, but dried fruit snacks are really just glorified candy. Because it still contains the fiber, dried fruit is better for your body than is juice, but because the water is gone, it becomes a highly concentrated sticky sugar, which can cause cavities very quickly. The occasional raisin or dried fruit is not much of a concern, but just be aware of their cavity-causing potential so that they are not eaten all day long. I try to keep them out of the house.

Crackers may show lots of complex carbohydrates listed on the nutrition label, but they convert to sugar easily because they are made with processed flour.

Hence, a cracker and piece of milk chocolate may have the same amount of available sugar for your teeth. One is considered "healthy" and the other one not, yet they would probably create cavities at the same rate based on their biochemical makeups. Who knows—crackers may even cause cavities more quickly because of the lower fat content!

Dark chocolate (70 percent or more cocoa) is relatively better for your teeth than milk chocolate. It has a higher fat content, lowering the sugar concentration. Even though dark chocolate is considered indulgent, bananas, oranges, fruit snacks, and crackers all have a greater capacity to cause cavities than does dark chocolate. Personally, I eat a little piece of dark chocolate every day as a midmorning snack. Delicious! If you want to indulge your child with a treat, don't feel guilty about 70 percent dark chocolate a few times a week. It is much better than a dried fruit snack!

Eating For Zero Cavities

Now that we have reviewed the food lists, below are the meal and snack options for a typical day in a zero-cavity household. It is generally assumed that your preschooler or young child will have crackers or pretzels at school once a day, so I recommend focusing more on what you do at home and with the foods you send to school with older children. Here is a summary of what a whole day would look like, for visual learners:

Options/Day in a Zero-Cavity Household	Drinks Are Always Whole Milk and Water Unless Indicated Otherwise. Water Should Be Offered at the End of Every Snack/Meal.
Breakfast	Oatmeal with applesauce and cinnamon (no sugar), shredded-wheat dry cereal with whole milk, smoothie (optional) with a water chaser, bacon or sausage, eggs, cheese, fresh fruit. Limit bananas and oranges to only one meal maximum.
Snack	Apples, cheese, reheated chicken, crunchy vegetables (steamed frozen works).
Lunch	Anything for main dish, with apples or carrots (with ranch dip) instead of crackers/pretzels, or applesauce instead of fruit snacks. If you think a sweet is necessary, keep it to once a week, offer 70 percent dark chocolate, or send school-aged children with money for ice cream, if available.
Snack	Celery with peanut butter, carrots with hummus, squares of whole-grain toast with 100 percent peanut butter, or pieces of chicken with frozen veggies.
Dinner	Any dinner item for main dish. Any dinner items for sides.
Dessert (optional)	Fresh fruit, ice cream, frozen yogurt, or 70 percent dark chocolate (drink water and brush teeth before bed).

When in doubt about whether a snack is bad for the teeth, use a stopwatch. Chew it yourself. Don't pick at it with your tongue. And check to see if it is still stuck on your teeth five minutes, seven minutes, or ten minutes later. If it is still on the teeth after seven minutes (assuming you don't pick at it with your tongue, which many children will not do), and it contains any carbohydrates, it is not good for the teeth. And if you can see it on the top surface of the teeth, imagine how long it will stay stuck *in between* the teeth! Who knows? You don't need a complicated, million-dollar, scientific study to figure this out. Don't take my word for it. You can be your own scientist. They have done studies on this before and found something surprising: most people are horrible at guessing what stays stuck on teeth. Nobody guessed that crackers were stickier than caramel, but it's unfortunately true.

More Chocolate, Fewer Crackers

The reason I make such a big deal about crackers is that they are the dictionary definition of *insidious* (according to *Merriam-Webster*): "Insidious: harmful but enticing. Of a disease: developing so gradually as to be well established before becoming apparent."

Every day, all across America, parents wonder how their four-year-olds have holes in their teeth. The cavity actually started years before, but now that the tooth is literally broken, it is too late for prevention. You don't have to let cavities sneak up on you. Once you label frequent cracker consumption as one of the major culprits of cavity formation, the solution to prevention becomes blaringly obvious. The extra brushing, extra fluoride, and even flossing recommended by most dentists (although all helpful) won't keep pace with frequent cracker consumption. Most children don't have weak enamel; they have too frequent consumption of processed flour snacks or natural liquid sugars, which have *caused* the weak enamel. Although weak enamel does exist, it is reported at about 1–3 percent of the population, and it usually presents in a distinct way, differently from normal cavities.

To put it simply, processed flour easily converts to sugars, creating the lactic acid that begins the cavity-forming process. It's an unexpected trap for parents who are concerned about the health of their children. Parents who are concerned about nutrition won't give kids candy all day long, but they may give whole-grain crackers all day long. Unfortunately for the teeth, the bacteria do not care whether the simple carbohydrate is supplied by candy or crackers. They get it either way. Cavities from processed starches happen more slowly than from sugar, undoubtedly, but they can happen nonetheless.

The reason your dentist may not have told you about this is because he would have sounded insane talking about this ten years ago. The old food pyramid had carbohydrates as a base. If we told parents to eat fewer crackers, it would have been blasphemy. But that old food pyramid didn't work out too well, and many researchers now know it was just wrong. Having a diet based on carbohydrates has increased the risk for obesity, diabetes, heart disease, and cavities. The problem is that people did not flock to more fruits and vegetables to get away from fats. They instead flocked to processed foods that aren't any better for you. Thankfully, with the recent trend away from processed foods and the allowance that fat can be acceptable nutritionally, dentists can finally start talking more about this without sounding completely crazy. Just a few months before this publication, eggs and cholesterol have been exonerated by the 2015–2020 US dietary guidelines. Less sugar is recommended. That is great news for teeth! It's going to take a while for us to change our habits, but we have to start today. Cavities do not care about the latest food craze. Fat, protein, and fiber do not cause cavities. Simple or processed carbohydrates do. No matter what is happening in the current nutritional debates, or future ones, this will remain true. Fat is a tooth's best friend, and teeth do not care what anyone else thinks.

Why More Chocolate?

Counterintuitively, your teeth would be better off if you had a small piece of 70 percent dark chocolate instead of a pretzel, a cracker, or even dried fruit. (I can't say the same for milk chocolate—sorry.) Dark chocolate has a higher fat content and therefore a lower carbohydrate concentration relative to crackers. It is similar to peanut butter that has some added sugar. Cavity-causing bacteria won't selectively only break down the sugars in chocolate; it must process the fat, too. Since it has to "wade through" all of the fat molecules, it will process the sugar a little more slowly.

My favorite is 70 percent dark chocolate. Dark chocolate in particular has more fat than it has sugar. In other words, fat is the majority of the mass, while sugar is a minority. The higher the cocoa concentration the better, because this increases the fat content and lowers the sugar content.

Dark chocolate also happens to contain some chemicals that may strengthen your enamel. Toothpaste manufacturer Theodent extracted a chemical from dark chocolate and used it to make toothpaste that has been shown to strengthen enamel. More research is needed, but it looks promising. I view it as one more excuse to eat dark chocolate. Now, don't go crazy and eat dark chocolate all day long. But you knew that already, right? I even give my three-year-old dark chocolate a few times a week (yet our house is cracker free!).

What about milk chocolate? Milk chocolate does not have the same health benefits as dark chocolate, but because of its higher fat content, it is better than most other candies (if you are going to have a piece of candy anyway). In other words, if you had a choice (for your teeth) between milk chocolate, a sucker, or a chewy fruity candy, choose the milk chocolate. The milk chocolate has less fat and more sugar than does dark chocolate (and no enamel-strengthening chemicals), but the sugar doesn't last as long as that of a hard sucker or chewy fruity candy. I wouldn't recommend milk chocolate every day because it lacks any health benefits dark chocolate may potentially provide, but I view crackers in the same way. I also do not recommend crackers every day, either. When you think of it that way, the average American family can usually get away with more chocolate than expected and should have significantly fewer crackers than expected when it comes to cavities. Have more chocolate and fewer crackers than you originally expected, and your teeth will be happier. My office gives out a piece of dark chocolate to every new family to drive this point home.

I have made my case for why crackers are bad for teeth (because of sticky, processed starch). Some dentists and doctors may argue against me for recommending dark chocolate. Let's pretend, for argument's sake, that I am somehow completely off base when it comes to dark chocolate and that crackers and dark chocolate both cause cavities at the same rate. This wouldn't be that surprising, because even apples and skim milk can cause cavities as well. Even if you don't like dark chocolate for teeth, it is still better than crackers because parents have an easier time saying no to chocolate. Biochemistry explains 20 percent of why chocolate is better for teeth, and psychology explains the other 80 percent. It is too easy to allow children to eat crackers all day because it is not candy. It is not that crackers are that inherently bad, it is the *habits* that they create and the fact that they are an extremely sticky starch. Even if crackers were vastly superior nutritionally to dark chocolate, they are still a sticky starch that can cause cavities when eaten in excess. Simply switch to whole-grain bread for similar nutrition without the stickiness.

As a parent concerned about the health of your child, you are not going to let your child eat dark chocolate (or even milk chocolate) all day long. That sounds absurd to a parent who is even somewhat concerned about nutrition. However, parents all across America and the world allow their children to graze on bite-size crackers (or other dry flour products, such as dry processed cereal) because it is considered *healthy* (as in not sweet). But if you want to prevent cavities, you should be more "afraid" of crackers than plain chocolate. As mentioned before, grazing on chocolate or crackers (or any other food with carbohydrates) is bad for teeth, so both should be given in limited amounts. Remember, frequency of exposure to simple carbohydrates is the biggest factor in cavity formation from a mathematical standpoint.

Ice Cream

I fully admit that I don't think we will be able to discover any amazing health benefits of ice cream. Wouldn't that be nice? Regardless, if you are going to have a dessert anyway, I recommend ice cream (or frozen yogurt) rather than other desserts when it comes to your teeth.

For teeth, ice cream, frozen yogurt, and regular yogurt are the same. They all have a lot of added sugar. When you have a small scoop of ice cream, you sit down, you eat it, you drink some water, and it is done. The ice cream rinses away quickly. It doesn't stay on your teeth for a long time, especially when you can have a sip of water afterward. If you're afraid of the sugar in ice cream for teeth, then you should be equally afraid of the sugar in store-bought yogurt, a smoothie, or fresh fruit. (Remember, we are not having a nutrition discussion here—that is another book.) Twenty minutes of acid is still twenty minutes of acid whether something is nutritious or not nutritious.

I have seen far too many families that strive for optimally healthy children avoid all excess sugars, but their children still end up with eight cavities because they gave them sticky, whole-grain starches all day. You don't have to cut all sugar in the diet to be cavity-free. Just be strategic about it if you do decide to include it.

However, I recommend that families add ice cream only if they take away something else. It would be counterproductive if you ate crackers or potato chips all day and then added the ice cream. So cut out the crackers, add vegetables, and then add the ice cream. Many parents like me enjoy giving their children an occasional dessert. If you do, ice cream beats a sucker or sticky candies any day of the week. It even beats a cracker because it doesn't get jammed between the teeth. If you are going to do dessert anyway, choose ice cream instead of a sucker or an ice pop, and drink a sip of water afterward.

Fresh fruit is, of course, the better dessert nutritionally, but for those of us who aren't perfect, stick with ice cream.

One final note: since my daughter is a dentist's kid, I admit to an irrational fear of my child turning into Willie Wonka from the 2005 movie *Charlie and the Chocolate Factory*. In the movie, the story suggests that Willie Wonka is inspired to own a candy factory because his dentist father never ever let him eat any candy. I try to offset this irrational fear by compromising with dark chocolate, ice cream, and going a little crazy with sweets only on vacations or for two days after Halloween. I believe in moderation in everything. And then I always make sure my kids have a drink of water after eating. Moral of the story: you don't have to be a crazy dentist dad to stay cavity-free.

PRINCIPLE ZERO: FLOSSING

PRINCIPLE ZERO: Floss when the teeth touch one another (but only the important ones).

Why do I not include flossing as a "real" principle? Because flossing is not *required* to prevent cavities. Despite every dentist's recommendation to floss (including mine), there is no strong evidence that flossing prevents cavities. If dentistry considers itself truly evidence based, then we must be willing to admit this when it comes to cavities. Please keep in mind that I still recommend that parents floss their child's teeth when they touch, but my argument is that we should look at diet as more important than flossing from an evidence-based perspective. There is evidence that frequency of food on the teeth affects cavities and that different diets can help prevent cavities, but not flossing. It sounds sacrilegious, but it is true.

If I was forced to choose between flossing and having no crackers in the house, I would choose keeping crackers and dry flour cereal out of the house every single time. The few times when parents told me they flossed their child's teeth religiously, yet still ended up with eight cavities, the story was always the same: their child was addicted to crackers. Out of one hundred families I interviewed who had cavity-free children, 99 percent gave their child crackers once a day or less on average. Only about half of the cavity-free kids had their teeth flossed. It was virtually impossible for me to find a child who was cavity-free at age five where the parents reported giving their child crackers three times a day or more.

Sometimes it isn't what you do. It is what you *don't* do.

As mentioned previously, younger siblings will consistently get multiple cavities even if older siblings had none. Is it likely that parents were flossing the oldest sibling's teeth but not flossing the younger siblings' teeth? Unlikely. In most instances, it would probably be floss all or floss none. What is more likely is that parents allow the younger sibling to graze on crackers more frequently (it keeps the younger kids quiet while parents attend to other children). This could easily explain how families have an older sibling with no cavities without having flossed and a younger sibling with multiple cavities. It wasn't the two suckers that younger one snuck in every month; it was the crackers he or she had three times a day for three years straight.

Flossing potentially only helps with mildly imperfect diets. It's similar to the saying for losing weight: you can't outexercise a bad diet. The same is true for teeth. You can't outfloss a bad diet. And you can't outbrush a bad diet. If your child eats candy or crackers all day, or drinks juice all day, flossing away the bacteria at night is not enough to compensate for the constant acid attacks that are produced from the frequent consumption of simple carbohydrates.

Flossing and brushing lessen the amount of bacteria that remain on teeth, but it is not realistic to completely eliminate all of the bacteria in your mouth, nor would it be logical to attempt it. There are also some good bacteria that you want to keep in your mouth. The mathematics of cavities also shows that the only way to keep acid to a minimum is to lower the frequency of carbohydrates. The thickness of the bacteria between the teeth is capped at a maximum variable. The frequency of carbohydrates in a day can range from zero to twenty-four hours.

Flossing most likely helps by a certain percentage, but what percentage (if any) is still to be determined. However, just as a dentist will have a hard time not recommending nightly brushing to remove the daily accumulation of bacteria, it is hard to imagine that leaving the bacteria to thrive in between the teeth for years would be helpful, either. Flossing helps you cover your bases in your goal for zero cavities for your child, and it makes up for inferior genetics (for teeth that touch early) or imperfections in diet (such as having pretzels at preschool), but it is not a cure-all.

Since your child is going to have pretzels at preschool, I recommend that you start flossing as soon as the teeth touch. If there is space in between the teeth, there is no need to floss because brushing can clean the bacteria.

To recap, flossing is not required for every child in order to achieve zero cavities, but it may be for your child. So, to ensure zero cavities, I recommend it when the teeth start to touch.

Tips for flossing:

1) Use the children's flossers unless you have amazing dexterity.
2) Reuse the flossers the way you reuse a toothbrush. A sample pack of three can last you six months. You wouldn't throw away a toothbrush every time you used it, would you?
3) To make your life easier, only floss the high-risk spots. The high-risk spots include the upper front teeth and the back molars if they are touching. It is much easier to explain flossing in video format, so visit TheDentistDad.com/flossing for a better visual explanation of the areas to floss and the areas you can skip.

IT'S NOT JUST FOR KIDS

Applying The Three Cavity-Prevention Principles To Teenagers And Adults

What you eat and the frequency of your meals and snacks are also the most important factors when it comes to cavity formation in teens and adults. And because teens and adults don't always consume an ideal diet, brushing, flossing, and fluoride become important tools to decrease the volume of bacteria that grow on and between teeth. Let's assume brushing is a given. (If you aren't even brushing your own teeth every day, I doubt you would have read this far.) I realize that half of those reading this book do not floss, yet not all of you get cavities every six months. Just as for kids, diet is more important than flossing.

For example, just like kids, if you eat crackers or pretzels all day long, flossing won't matter. If you eat a smoothie for breakfast, a sandwich with an apple for lunch, and chicken with rice and vegetables for dinner every day, and you have water between meals, you most likely can get away without ever flossing and still not get cavities. (I don't recommend trying this, but every dentist has patients who get away with not flossing. Ask my wife.) However, as soon as you add pretzels to the afternoon snack routine every day, then, suddenly, flossing becomes a helpful cavity-prevention tool.

Everyone has a different limit of what they can get away with, which is partially based on genetics. Here are a few examples from teenagers and parents I have talked with who got surprise cavities. You will notice that following the three principles would have prevented cavities in all of the examples.

1. A teenager went from zero to eleven cavities in six months. She cried when I broke the news to her. She was in a "running start program" (college classes while still in high school) and drinking

sweetened ice tea all day long. If she had the sweet tea just at lunch, she probably would have been fine.

2. A college student decided he wanted to be healthier, so he went on an all-organic juice diet. Instead of having juice at certain times with water in between, he sipped on it all day long. Zero to eight cavities in six months.

3. A father of a three-year-old with cavities worked at an established gaming software company near Seattle. His company provided unlimited beverages and snacks, which he took advantage of frequently throughout the day. Since starting to work there, he has had a lot of cavity issues, and he didn't realize this until I reviewed the principles with him to prevent more cavities in his daughter.

4. A college student moved to Britain. Though she had never had a cavity her entire life, after a few months of drinking sweetened hot tea throughout the day, she suddenly had several cavities.

What is the common thread in all of these examples? Frequency. The teeth of teens and adults would be better off if they drank thirty-two ounces of soda in a five-minute period rather than sipping on something organically sweet all day long. (You will have some major health issues if you drink thirty-two ounces of soda every day in five minutes, but your teeth will survive if it is done quickly.)

Adults And Root Caries

Treating adults is not my expertise, but I will briefly review a few key differences between children and older adults.

According to studies, adults over sixty years old have a greater prevalence of cavities on the roots in select demographics. This happens when gums recede and the roots lack the tougher enamel coverage. Once the dentin is exposed, it is more susceptible to the acid attack by bacteria, especially since dentin demineralizes with less acid exposure than does enamel. Based on the greater susceptibility of the root, people with a lot of gum recession would need to be more wary of all sources of carbohydrates—not just the stickier ones—compared to a child, whose roots are not exposed. The three principles still apply to those with gum recession, but you may have to adjust meals to include fewer instances of easily digestible carbohydrates or immediately brush after these meals with fluoride toothpaste. I don't have anecdotal evidence for adults, but the prevention principles should carry over on a theoretical basis.

Also, keep in mind that I need to prevent cavities in my patient base for only about ten years to be considered cavity-free. Family dentists have to go decades.

I would argue an adult dentist's challenge is five times harder, considering that time is the biggest variable.

Additionally, if you are taking medications, check with your dentist to see if dry mouth can be a side effect. Dry mouth, whether caused by medication or other issues, can wreak havoc on teeth because there isn't enough saliva to rinse away the acid after meals or to supply the minerals that remineralize the teeth. Talk to your dentist about fluoride trays and rinses, dry-mouth rinses, xylitol gum, or other methods to try to help compensate for this.

Uncontrolled acid reflux can be a major problem as well, as it puts acid on the teeth without any carbohydrates. Work with your medical doctor to get your acid reflux under control, and talk with your dentist about extra preventive steps you can take.

Remember that unsweetened beverages are OK for teeth, but adding any carbohydrates means you should limit the time on teeth. Even just a plain latte has sugars from milk. For your teeth's sake, it is better to add a shot of syrup and drink it in twenty minutes than to sip on the milk latte for eight hours. You may have a different outcome for your gut, but we are talking teeth.

Part IV

Common Questions And Other Pediatric Dental Topics

EMOTIONAL INTELLIGENCE AND CAVITY PREVENTION: CAN YOU HAVE RULES AND EMPATHY AT THE SAME TIME?

One of the most common statements I hear is:

"My child won't let me brush his teeth."

Other common phrases include:

"I can't keep her from drinking juice all day."
"There is no way I will get her to stop eating crackers."

Beliefs like those stated above will obviously interfere with preventing cavities. Addressing these common statements brings up the touchy subject of parenting philosophies and limit setting. I am not writing a parenting book. My only purpose is to prevent cavities. However, preventing cavities requires setting limits in order to have healthy teeth. Teeth do not care about parenting styles, and neither do I. Many parents want some specific, practical tips on how to set limits without being overly harsh. So I will discuss some resources that many parents have found helpful, and you can decide what works best for your child. If you can find a way to set healthy limits with other methods, great! I truly believe there is not one perfect way for every family, but I do want parents with different parenting styles to "get along." Even with my own three daughters, my wife and I have had to be flexible. What worked with one kid doesn't always work with next kid. I find that even my own "parenting style" changes with time.

If you have a strong-willed child (or an uncooperative brusher or eater) and need some good parenting books, my recommendations are: *How to Raise an Emotionally Intelligent Child*, *Love and Logic Magic for Early Childhood*, and *1-2-3 Magic: Effective Discipline for Children 2–12*.

Since we are going to talk about limit setting and empathy, we need to discuss emotional intelligence and emotion coaching. First, I will give a brief description of what emotion coaching is, and then give some examples on how to use it to keep your child's teeth healthy at the end. You may or may not be very familiar with emotion coaching already. Let's review what emotional intelligence is before we relate it to preventing cavities. Regardless of your children's willfulness or cooperativeness, emotional intelligence is an important skill to help them develop. To understand emotional intelligence, I highly recommend reading the book *How to Raise an Emotionally Intelligent Child* by John Gottman, PhD, founder of the Gottman Institute. If you read only one book on parenting, this is the book I would recommend because Dr. Gottman's research is much more scientifically thorough than many other books you may find. Dr. Gottman is one of the leading experts on marriage stability and emotion coaching. In his research, he found that children who had parents who used emotion coaching techniques had lower rates of infections, higher test scores, and better social skills. In my observations, some parents are very big proponents of emotional intelligence, but many have not read "the book," or any book, on emotional coaching. These parents are often doing well, but they may leave out important and helpful details that Dr. Gottman has uncovered through his research.

The nice thing about emotion coaching is that the focus is not on discipline. Previous parenting philosophies widely taught from the 1950s on focused solely on discipline. Gottman's emotion coaching focuses on having an emotional connection with your child.

Personally, I welcome this change, and evidence shows it is more effective at raising children with higher emotional intelligence quotients, or "EQs." Emotion coaching may seem confusing at first because the focus is not on discipline, but that does not mean that there is no limit setting. Setting limits based on your family's values is still very important. Creating the emotional connection is important, but it loses effectiveness without limit setting. According to Dr. Gottman's research, children who are raised without limit setting can become rather aggressive.

The final step in emotion coaching is problem solving when kids breech the limits. You work with your child to figure out how to stay within the set limits in the future even though the child may be feeling strong emotions. For example, your family likely has a rule (limit) about not hitting others even when the child is angry, frustrated, or jealous. Dr. Gottman states that all emotions are acceptable, but not all behavior is acceptable. Being angry with someone is OK, but hitting that person is not OK. When the child hits, then you problem solve with the child to figure out what to do instead of hitting the next time he or she is upset.

From an oral health and cavity prevention standpoint, it is no different when it comes to emotions and behaviors. All emotions are acceptable, but not all behaviors are acceptable. When you change your family values to make having healthy teeth a priority, everything else falls into place. All of a sudden, brushing your teeth every night is not negotiable; it happens no matter what. Your child can be frustrated because he doesn't want to brush his teeth. You can help him use his words to explain his frustration, but brushing still has to be done. Additionally, drinking juice all day just never happens. Your toddler can be angry that she can't have juice whenever she wants, but she learns that because we want to have healthy teeth, we don't have juice every day. Your family values determine where you draw the line in the sand. Where you draw that line differs from family to family. If your family values include good oral health, you follow the prevention principles.

The good news about emotion coaching and preventing cavities is that you don't have to be perfect. According to Dr. Gottman, if you are emotion coaching 40 percent of the time, you are doing a pretty good job. So, if one night you "flip your lid" and brush your child's teeth while you are really angry, it's not the end of the world. In fact, it gives you an opportunity to model how to apologize. "I am sorry I was angry last night when I brushed your teeth. It just makes me feel frustrated when you are whining and crying while I brush your teeth. I feel much happier when you choose to be a good helper, and I want to help you do that. Perhaps I'm hurting you. Is there one spot that bugs you when I brush? Should I be more gentle? Thanks for letting me know that spot bugs you. We can practice stretching your cheeks so I can brush that spot more easily."

Some parents may feel they don't have the power to change habits in their children. This is not true. It all depends on what is important to you. The habit simply has to be a family value that's strong enough to put into practice consistently. For example, if you drink red wine, you have a rule that your child doesn't drink red wine. Of course, you would argue, no parent who values health would allow a child to drink wine. That is my point. Every parent, no matter his parenting philosophy, has the intrinsic capability of enforcing a rule. Your child may want to drink red wine or run into a fire at a campground. He may want to grab the hot stove or run across the street. But you will stop him. You may not talk about the rules all day or post them anywhere, but you enforce them nonetheless. You just have to think they are important enough.

Many parents of two- or three-year-olds in my practice will say things like, "I can't keep her from drinking juice all day," or "There is no way I will get her to stop her cracker habit." When parents say this, they actually believe it to be true, so they are not capable of changing their children's habits. However, once you realize that you have the intrinsic capability of keeping things from your child, there is no excuse anymore. And after a series of experiments that may last for minutes, hours, days, or (for a two-year-old) months, children will learn what they can and can't get away with. Kids are extremely smart. It is OK to set limits based on your family's values. If you want zero cavities, you can set up limits to achieve a healthy mouth that resists cavities.

If your child is frustrated over a rule such as cooperating with brushing, it's OK to say, "I'm sorry you're frustrated, but the rule in our house is that we have to brush our teeth to keep them healthy. Would you like to pick out another toothbrush?" If he still refuses (which some kids will), then use different techniques. However, you still consistently keep the rule of brushing one's teeth.

Dr. Gottman recommends looking for opportunities to say yes. When it comes to cavity prevention and other healthy habits, you also want to avoid opportunities where you have to say no. My theory is that every parent has a limited number of times that he can say no in a day before he goes a little crazy. I base this purely on personal experience. Once you go a little crazy, it is easy to give in. If there is not a compelling family value to not give in, or you also have an older sibling to take care of, it sometimes becomes easier to give in. So instead of saying no all day, plan ahead. Don't buy the juice or crackers in the first place. If you have juice boxes at eye level, you are asking for whining. If they are hidden in the garage, you have a better chance. Regarding snack foods, it starts at the grocery store. If it is not in the house, you reduce the chance for whining at home.

It is better to have one tantrum in the grocery store than seven tantrums every day. So if your toddler asks for something very sugary at the store, it's OK to set limits. If it makes you feel better, even Dr. Gottman states that there are certain circumstances where emotion coaching cannot be accomplished effectively. One such time is a tantrum in a grocery store. You simply have to get out of the situation and save emotion coaching for a more socially acceptable time. (Hint: stay away from the candy and juice sections of the store.)

MY CHILD PREFERS CRACKERS OVER OTHER FOODS

I can't tell you how many times parents have told me, "My child prefers crackers over other foods. She is a very picky eater." There is a very good biochemical reason for this.

If you give most human children a choice between a cracker and something else that's considered healthy, they will almost always choose the cracker. Why? Because the cracker is processed into flour, and that flour turns to sugar easily while sitting on the tongue. Once sugar is on the tongue, the brain receives a pleasure signal from dopamine. This is the same neurotransmitter that is associated with some drug addictions. The brain says,

"Give me more!" We, as humans, are hardwired to crave sugar, most likely because it wasn't always available so easily. This is the same reason that whenever my wife makes a batch of brownies, I seem to eat the entire plate without stopping.

So when a parent says that his son is a picky eater who prefers crackers, he's saying that the child's dopamine receptors are working perfectly and the food companies did a great job in making their products desirable. In other words, you, as a parent, have to make the decision for them to not eat crackers.

My own daughter said it best while we were on vacation one summer. She was five years old, and, as you have guessed, she doesn't eat crackers on a regular basis. We had a popular brand with us on vacation, when I usually throw caution to the wind nutritionally. (This is also when we have other sugary treats on a short-term basis.) My daughter was saying things like, "These crackers are my favorite snack." The best thing she told me was, "Dad, once I start eating these, I can't stop." I laughed out loud when I heard this. My daughter was old enough to verbalize what every two-year-old's brain is thinking. Crackers are very addicting.

If you do need to stop a current habit, keep in mind that it may take a few days for blood sugar levels to stabilize. Think of how often the blood sugar is spiking during the day every time crackers are consumed. When you switch to foods that don't spike the blood sugar as much, there may be a day or two of crankiness until the body adjusts.

As you can see, you will make your life much easier by keeping crackers out of the house. Many parents have done this arbitrarily for years. Why can't you do it with a conscious decision to keep sticky starches off your child's teeth and cut down on whining at the same time?

JUST TELL ME WHAT TO DO

For those of you who would prefer simple directives instead of the explanation behind them, here is what I do, in no particular order:

Follow the three prevention principles:

1) Help your child brush for twenty seconds every night, with only water after that.
2) Give your child five or six organized minimeals a day, with water in between.
3) Give your child snack foods that prevent cavities or that don't cause them quickly.

Have smoothies (with fiber) instead of juice. Limit smoothies to once or twice a day at most. Have a sip of water afterward.

Have oatmeal, shredded-wheat cereal, or bacon and eggs for breakfast instead of dry-flour cereal.

Anytime you would consider giving apple juice, give applesauce instead.

It's better to send ice cream, pudding or 70 percent dark chocolate into your child's lunch instead of crackers. Crackers are stickier than you think. It's better to have sugar quickly than starches that are sticky.

Have water with every meal, even if there is a milk or smoothie present as well.

Have your child eat as much candy as she wants for a day or two after Halloween or Valentine's Day, and then get rid of it all. Or eat it yourself.

If you have a son, help him brush his teeth for twenty seconds every night until he is eighteen years old. OK, this isn't necessary for every boy—but it is for a few.

If you have a daughter, help her brush her teeth for twenty seconds every night until she is six or seven—unless you need to help for longer.

Don't let any child brush on his or her own unless you check things for a few nights to make sure he or she is doing an adequate job.

You can scrape the child's teeth gently with a toothpick to check for plaque. If plaque (that soft white stuff) is still on the teeth anywhere, show the child how to get it or keep helping.

Once children are brushing on their own, that's when you want to enforce the two-minutes-twice-a-day rule.

Let your children eat crackers at preschool when other parents bring them. Don't let them eat them at home or pack them in lunches.

For your children's teeth, it is better to have ice cream every night than it is to have crackers three times a day.

Suckers are still horrible for teeth. Save them for airplane rides or car trips over four hours.

For potty training, buy xylitol suckers online and use them only while potty training. They may help prevent cavities instead of causing them during that time.

Try to cut out multiple nighttime feedings as close to twelve months as possible for teeth's sake.

Ask your mother-in-law to give your kids ice cream and chocolate instead of hard candies or crackers.

Try to substitute string cheese, precut apple slices, applesauce packets, and bread pr oducts for dried crackers or dried fruit for on-the-go snacks whenever possible. (You can download a shopping list of over 50 snack ideas that I approve at TheDentistDad.com/shoppinglist.)

If your child is very sick and you are worried about hydration, give her apple juice and Pedialyte nonstop as needed for a few days. As soon as she's better, make sure to switch back to water and put up with a day of fussing.

Scientific studies have shown that limit setting is an important part of emotion coaching. Setting limits based on having a healthy body and healthy teeth is the right thing to do as a parent. All emotions are acceptable, but not all behavior is acceptable.

The number-one thing you can do for your children:

Make sure they associate being thirsty with drinking water.

Keeping crackers out of the house is a close second.

WHAT SHOULD I DO WITH DAY CARE, PRESCHOOL, NANNIES, AND IN-LAWS?

Let's address each one separately.

Nannies/Babysitters: Talking with nannies should theoretically be the easiest because it is an employer-employee relationship. Explain what you have learned, print out the snack guide, and review my principles. Support the nanny with good shopping habits.

Day Care/Preschool: Although technically this is an employer-employee relationship, it's a little more difficult to deal with because the day care also takes care of other children. Although hours may vary, I will treat day cares and preschools in the same category. Thankfully, most well-run day cares already have organized snack times. This is a requirement of any day care I would leave my kids with, and I would switch day cares if they aren't willing to keep snack times organized.

Juice is a little more common, unfortunately. Given the fact that juice is widely known to be a cavity causer, I don't think it has any place in any day care or preschool setting (other than smoothies for breakfast, with a sip of water afterward, as I have discussed earlier). I feel so strongly about this that you should feel free to download a letter I have written and give it to your day care or pre-school. They can talk with me directly if you don't want to talk with them. Please ask them if they can switch to applesauce instead of juice first, but if you need help, download the letter at TheDentistDad.com/letters.

As far as crackers go, that is going to be harder to change in the day care setting. My child's preschool has a snack similar to crackers maybe once a day. Since we don't have those snacks at home, that is only three or four times a week. I wouldn't worry about three or four times a week. That amount may be what flossing is for. However, if it is more than once a day, I would be more worried. This is usually in a day care setting and not pre-school. School inherently needs organized snack times, which is a good thing. When asking anyone to change to a healthier habit, remember to offer solutions instead of simply complaining. Bread or bagels are just as easy as crackers but not as sticky. Feel free to use the letters at theDentistDad.com/letters. To be honest, sometimes it is better for a teacher to hear it from a doctor so you aren't the one sounding crazy. These are the people taking care of your child. You want to be as nice as possible. Feel free to pretend that you just thought the letter was interesting but it's not a big deal if it is hard to switch. Just spreading the message is helpful because most people don't know. Let them make the decision to make the switch, even if it was you who brought attention to it.

Grandparents and In-Laws: Dealing with relatives can often be the most difficult conversation, especially if it is your own parents! With all due respect to my wonderful in-laws, common thought processes are: "You turned out OK, and I did this with you." Again, focus on offering solutions and not on making their lives more difficult. Bread instead of crackers. Have ice cream every night on one condition: no more crackers. This is my personal favorite, because your mother- or father-in-law can now still "spoil" the grandchildren, but you can avoid the cavities. Just as I recommend earlier, use dark chocolate as the occasional sweet instead of hard candies. All parents everywhere have a difficult time taking advice from someone whose diapers they had to change. Be as gentle as possible with their ego. Make sure to start off and finish with how grateful you are, and let them have fun with dark chocolate and ice cream in moderation if they cut back on the sticky starches. My letter written to day care providers can be used as well.

WHAT ABOUT VISITING FRIENDS?

Let's say I have done a more-than-adequate job of motivating you to go for zero cavities. You have thrown out all the crackers. Juice is forbidden in your household. String-cheese packets and precut apple slices are stored in the fridge. You actually floss four spots every night in your child's teeth.

Then your daughter goes to a birthday party (cue the dramatic music) where soda is being served. Should you grab the table, throw it up into the air so that the soda spills all over the three-year-olds, yell at the top of your lungs, "You are a horrible parent who lacks dental and health education!" grab your child, and run away? Of course not!

Birthday parties may take you out of your carefully constructed zero-cavity household, but that doesn't mean your child can't enjoy the sweets that day. Our goal is not perfection. Nobody is perfect. Even if your goal is zero cavities, it is not achieved by perfection but instead by long-term consistency over a five-year period. Everyday habits are more important than occasional sugar splurges.

Having a soda at a birthday party is not going to ruin your child. As they say in *Frozen*, "Let it go." Since you don't have soda at home, there is a high chance your child won't like it anyway. Assuming you don't go to parties every day, a rule that you can have soda at parties is one that can still allow for zero cavities. It's not as if apple juice or organic fresh-squeezed lemonade is any better for your teeth. You don't get cavities from one day; you get them from everyday habits. If your child starts asking for it at home, simply explain that soda is a special treat for birthday parties and when going to the movies, but we don't have it at home because it would cause too many sugar bugs (or cavities).

TEACHERS GIVING OUT CANDY

This is a tough one because I am married to a teacher. The problem with teachers and candy is frequency. If one teacher hands out candy once a week, that is fine in my book. But if four teachers hand it out once a day, it becomes a problem. It is not the individual decision that is a problem but the cumulative effect. I would probably intervene only if this were happening more than once a week (unless it is dark chocolate, of course—then every day would be fine). If you feel you need to discuss this with the teacher or administration, be as nice as possible and give as many concrete examples as possible: "My son received six Jolly Ranchers in the last two weeks. I feel that the little bits of candy here and there are adding up to too much." Offer a compromise of 70 percent dark chocolate treats instead, or perhaps ice cream. Maybe even offer to buy the dark chocolate. This could start a conversation about how cavities really work. Let teachers and administrators borrow this book and then go out for martinis (or smoothies, or coffee, or whatever). This is how to be social and still worry about teeth.

I also have empathy for the other side of the spectrum. I'm not proposing having no candy ever, but, rather, something in the middle. If you control your home environment very well and don't have sweet snacks (other than dark chocolate or ice cream) more than once a week, then when your child gets a treat during social situations, it is not a big deal at all. As a pediatric dentist, I want to say this for the record. I am more worried about my child eating crackers three times a day at home than getting candy at school occasionally.

SPECIAL HEALTH-CARE NEEDS

Children with special health-care needs are statistically at higher risk for forming cavities. Unfortunately, there is not an easy answer to this. Zero cavities may not be attainable in some cases. But by being aware of how cavities are formed, you can adopt preventive measures to lessen or delay cavities. It is important to at least think about cavity prevention (in conjunction with instructions from your medical doctor) so that cavities don't turn into an additional problem to address. Pain from cavities can create their own issues, such as trouble with eating. Give prevention your best effort, and talking with your dentist about any tips she may have will help. The hope, of course, is to try to prevent having an additional surgery for treating the cavities that grow too quickly. If medical recommendations make this impossible, you can at least start planning ahead.

THE CHILD IS NOT GAINING WEIGHT

If your doctor recommends that your child drink weight-gaining drinks throughout the day (which does not happen very frequently), this is a tough problem. If at all possible, still try to have the drinks or food every two to three hours, and try for as many sips of water as possible in order to rinse away any sugars and acids after every time your child drinks other liquids. Try to be creative. For more calories, add fats wherever you can, such as flaxseed oil to smoothies, peanut butter or other nut butters to smoothies, or even peanut butter with ice cream after dinner. Sneak vegetables into everything. Throw a little olive oil or grass-fed butter on the top of anything you can. Be creative. Schedule a visit with a registered dietician if you haven't done so already. She will have more time to discuss food options than will a medical doctor or dentist, and she may have a few more tricks up her sleeve as well. Make sure to ask if she has experience working with children who are picky eaters. If you don't find your dietician is helpful, don't be afraid to seek another opinion.

CHILDREN WHO NEED MEDICATION MORE THAN ONCE A DAY, INCLUDING ASTHMA MEDICATION

Some children, such as those with seizure disorders or asthma, need to take medicine that contains sugar more than once a day. Obviously, you need to curtail the seizures or asthma attacks, but what do you do about all that sugar? If at all possible, take the medication with a meal, and always offer a drink of water after every dose. Make it a game if you need to, but focus on water to rinse the sugars away. And still ensure an excellent brushing every twenty-four hours before bedtime.

SENSORY PROCESSING DISORDERS

Parents have been trying to get their children to eat their broccoli since the dawn of time. Broccoli aside, some children are pickier eaters than most. For most children, a few visits with a dietician and some extra work can be very effective. (Eating just one more vegetable a day is a good start.) While many children are not truly picky eaters (they're simply addicted to easily digestible carbohydrates because they are so sweet), there is a subset of children who have a diagnosed sensory processing disorder, which is more than just a preference for sweet things. You are most likely already seeing an occupational therapist, so make sure to ask about tips for brushing. And if at all possible, switch from crackers to foods that are better for the teeth. Ideally, you can get to the point where crackers and other sticky foods are not in the house and other healthy snacks can be tolerated. It is helpful to work toward this specific goal with your occupational therapist. Every little bit helps. The feel of a toothbrush. Water. Healthy foods. Depending on the severity of the sensory issues, this can be one of the toughest medical issues for cavity prevention. Unfortunately, subsequent treatment is also difficult because children with sensory issues usually do not tolerate dental treatment as well.

AUTISM SPECTRUM DISORDER

There is absolutely no one-size-fits-all solution with children with autism, especially given the range within autism spectrum disorder. My advice focuses on the milder end of the spectrum.

Because many children with autism often have sensory processing issues as well, fixing cavities in these children presents a unique set of challenges. The easiest cavities to fix are the ones that never appear. So focusing on the prevention principles in this book is the best place to start. If you haven't found a pediatric dentist yet, I would recommend trying one. Pediatric dentists tend to see a higher percentage of children with autism because of our extra training.

Many parents have told me that they see a noticeable difference in their children when they consume a gluten-free diet, but others don't see any difference at all. If you have chosen a gluten-free diet (for whatever reason), the silver lining that makes up for the inconvenience is that you avoid wheat flour. So when you are stressing about how much harder it is to have gluten-free snacks on hand, take solace in the fact that you are most likely choosing good-for-your-teeth snacks as well. It is not the gluten that poses the biggest cavity-causing risk from crackers, but the fact that crackers are easy to eat so frequently (although some argument could be made that the gluten makes the crackers "stickier"). If your child loves only crackers, start working with an occupational therapist as soon as possible to help with the ASD-associated sensory issues when it comes to food.

Autism spectrum disorder is often associated with sensory issues. There are many red flags you can screen for, as early as six months. For more information, I recommend autismspeaks.org; look for "Learn the Signs."

CONSIDER EXTRA FLUORIDE

The AAPD guidelines also recommend in-office prescription fluoride applications every three months for children at high risk for cavities. I prefer the topical application of fluoride versus the systemic fluoride. While diet is more important than fluoride, the fluoride definitely helps because diets can't be perfect. If your child has special needs and preventing cavities is going to be more difficult than average, then strongly consider starting fluoride treatments as early as age one. I recommend more frequent applications until children are able to rinse and spit out an over-the-counter fluoride rinse such as ACT Kids Anticavity Fluoride Rinse or Listerine Smart Rinse for Kids, or until they can sit in the chair and have a filling put in—whichever comes first. Please keep in mind these are my personal preferences, so talk to your dentist about his preferences and your unique situation.

GENERAL ADVICE FOR GETTING YOUR CHILD READY FOR THE DENTIST

Do bring in your child early and often. If you haven't already had your child's one-year exam, it is not too late. Remember that most one-, two-, and three-year-olds will cry for the brief visual exam. You don't have to worry about the cleaning part until they are ready. If they happen to sit for it, it makes for wonderful pictures. Under age three, the visual screening exam and the information your dentist can give you are more important than a professional cleaning.

Not every dentist focuses on prevention as proactively as I do (although a large majority do), but I will admit that this book goes into more detail than I have time for on any exam, or even over several exams. It's why I wrote it. This book contains everything I wish I could tell parents but don't have time to say. My focus is also mostly on diet above all else, whereas traditional thinking is to focus on dozens of other variables first. The other variables are helpful, but diet and frequency outweigh every other variable in my new paradigm.

In my office, if a one-year-old is low risk for cavities, we recommend a yearly checkup until age three. If we determine there is higher risk for cavities, we may recommend every three months or six months, depending on the level of concern. Teaching parents my prevention principles before bad habits start is the most effective prevention regime available. The visit at age one is 80 percent about teaching prevention principles and 20 percent about screening for high-risk areas. Of course, I had to do a lot of research to come up with my specific prevention principles, which are, I believe, more effective because they are based on biochemistry and math. While many veteran dentists have figured out crackers are bad for your teeth, it isn't necessarily common knowledge yet. If your dentist isn't convinced that diet is the secret to cavity prevention, let them know about my book. They can also get more articles and ask questions at TheDentistDad.com/dentists. I will try to answer every question, within reason. My goal is to help as many people as possible. I spent over three years researching journals to convince myself that my advice would hold up to the science. It does.

If a dentist has experience with infant exams, she can often spot a cavity before it starts (unless it is in between the teeth). Teeth that touch increase cavity risk, so dentists can point out that teeth are touching at an early age for that particular child and recommended flossing at an earlier age. At about age three, most children's back teeth start to touch, which allows the flour to start getting stuck between the teeth. Therefore, we switch to six-month exams in my office after age three even for kids at low risk for cavities. This enables us to get a head start on getting kids used to the dentist and to continue prevention strategies.

Coming in early also allows many children to get the crying out of the way so they can be cooperative by age four or five. From my perspective, many kids who have a first visit to the dentist at age four or five cry just as much, if not more, than the children who start visiting the office as infants or toddlers. My theory is that kids are afraid of getting vaccines. But in a strange twist, after going home a few times without getting a vaccine and with a toy in hand, kids start to like the dentist more than the pediatrician. So if your dentist does not see children under the age of three, find a pediatric dentist who does, and look for one who focuses on prevention. By not taking children under the age of three, that dentist is clearly stating that he has not learned any proactive approaches about prevention that he can teach you, and he's not following the current guidelines. Feel free to send such dentists my way so I can try to change their minds, because they are probably still really excellent doctors in other avenues.

While dentists (including me) were not taught my prevention principles in dental school, this does not discredit all of the other prevention tools we were taught. Every dentist knows that drinking juice all day or sucking on oranges all day is horrible for your teeth. Dentists already know not to eat or drink all day long. My goal is to add to the discussion that crackers are also horrible for teeth. Even more importantly, diet and frequency trump everything else in cavity prevention. My hope is that in the future, an approach to cavity prevention that is first based on diet will be common knowledge. However, always keep in mind that cavity prevention is 80 percent habits and only 20 percent knowledge. And good habits, as you now know, can start at age one.

Don't be concerned if your infant, toddler, or child cries for the brief exam. Tears will subside when she gets a sticker or a toy or perhaps sees other fun things. Focus more on the fun things. Distraction is an excellent technique for toddlers.

Additionally, you might consider buying a mirror (or ask your dentist if he or she has any disposable ones or old ones) and practice using it at home. Get your children used to the feel of it in their mouths so it is not a completely foreign object. Play dentist and have your kids practice lying down on the couch or floor while using the mirror. Keep in mind that even if you try all these things, and even if a child is excited about going to the next appointment, many young ones will still cry during the exam. Then, magically, around age four and a half, many kids will finally sit in the chair without crying. Yes, there are some kids who are absolutely amazing and will be fine before that age, but don't let it stop the kids with age-appropriate behavior from getting screened for early warning signs of cavities or parents from getting other useful prevention tips. Plus, it is often very helpful to get reinforcement from an authority figure such as the dentist to support your rule about brushing every night. Most kids will be nervous the first few times at a new place, anyway. Better to get it over with at age one instead of age five.

FLUORIDE REDUCES CAVITIES

My view on fluoride is slightly different from the ADA's recommendations. If you view diet and frequency (amount of time food is on teeth) as very important cavity-prevention strategies, you can be more conservative with fluoride.

The ADA's recommendations are based on broad public health policy. If I can't teach a parent about prevention principles by the child's first birthday, then the parent should follow all of the ADA's advice because fluoride is a very helpful medicine that can lessen the severity of cavities.

However, as you now know, what a child eats and drinks and how often the child does so are more important than fluoride. Let's talk about how fluoride can be helpful.

Fluoride works two in ways: topically and systemically. A topical application of fluoride makes tooth enamel more resistant to acid attacks by bacteria. Systemic fluoride in drinking water provides developing teeth with fluoride as they form.

Fluoridated water (in the correct amount) has been shown to reduce the amount of cavities. What is harder to prove, or is not certain, is whether the benefit comes from the topical effect of the drinking water rinsing over the teeth or from the systemic effect of swallowing fluoride so that it helps in forming teeth. The evidence keeps pointing toward the topical effect being the more important of the two. Since side effects seem to result from systemic fluoride, I lean more toward topical applications rather than systemic ones. With my daughter, I use as little toothpaste as possible because I know she swallows whatever we use (making it systemic).

And because I want zero cavities and no needles for my daughter, I also apply a topical prescription fluoride twice a year in the dental office. This provides the greatest cavity-prevention benefit with the least risk of possible side effects.

Topical fluoride comes from toothpaste, fluoride mouth rinse, prescription fluoride applications at the dentist (which are one hundred times as strong as toothpaste), or the fluoridated drinking water that rinses over the teeth as you drink it.

I decided to use prescription fluoride (in the dental office) on my children's teeth twice a year starting at age two because they eat crackers at preschool and we eat things with flour and sugar in them. Now, if you and your children have the "perfect tooth diet," they avoid all processed foods, have more vegetables than fruit, eat no grains, and drink water all day, then you probably don't need any fluoride to prevent cavities. (Keep in mind those are all big ifs, and it's just my opinion.) However, if your child's diet does contain processed foods, fluoride has been shown, over and over again, to help reduce cavities. I don't think you should give up on fluoride completely unless you cut out processed foods completely as well. It is just not very practical, especially with multiple kids and one or two parents having to work.

However, while fluoride is beneficial, too much can be a bad thing (as can any vitamin or medicine). Most people use too much toothpaste. I greatly restrict the amount of fluoride for my child by not using it before their back teeth are touching. For children under five, I recommend using fluoride toothpaste only once a day with a rice-size (versus pea-size) amount of toothpaste, to reduce potential fluoride intake. This is the same as the ADA guidelines. You can switch to a pea-size amount after age six or seven. This greatly reduces the risk of fluorosis on the developing secondary (adult) teeth but still provides the anticavity benefit. If your child eats crackers three times a day, he or she should brush three times a day with a pea-size amount of fluoride toothpaste to help compensate for the diet. While that is a viable option, I think cutting back on crackers is preferable (and takes less effort if you start the correct snack habits early).

Too Little Fluoride Is A Problem. Too Much Fluoride Is A Problem.

Let's discuss the documented risks of too much fluoride. If a child chronically ingests twice the amount of recommended fluoride, mild fluorosis can occur. The teeth form normally, and they are rock hard or very resistant to decay, but they have little white mottled spots on them. This is a mild side effect, but it would be ideal to avoid it, especially in the front permanent teeth, for aesthetic reasons. To help avoid this, I would try to prevent cavities by following my three principles start-ing at age one and not using fluoride toothpaste until the baby molars are all in (usually by age two or three). Once you do use fluoride toothpaste, use as little as possible. A rice-size smear is plenty (and I literally mean the size of a grain of rice). Swipe the toothbrush over the tube rather than squeezing the tube. By delaying fluoride toothpaste, you decrease the risk of fluorosis. If you start to use it when the back teeth touch, you start getting the benefit from it when it really becomes important. In my mind, this is a good compromise for those who are also focusing on diet at the same time and do not have other risk factors. Remember that hav-ing multiple feedings at night after age 18 months is a risk factor for cavities.

The current ADA guidelines recommend starting fluoride at age one. But the cavity rate in children is not going down considerably despite this recommendation. I contend this is because the ADA is still focused on the old paradigm (more drugs to prevent a disease). For parents of children in my practice, my three prevention principles are working. I contend they are more effec-tive (and safer) than more or earlier fluoride. However, early fluoride is still a good recommendation as public health policy because the general public is often not focused on prevention through diet, nor will they take the time to read an entire book about it. In other words,

I agree with the ADA when it comes to their policy for public health, but not for every individual family or my own family. I would support a statement along the lines of "Start fluoride toothpaste at different ages depending on your child's risk factor for cavities based on habits and diet." That guideline would be more accurate, in my opinion, but extremely vague and harder to follow. The ADA already recommends varying frequency of fluoride applications in the office based on caries risk, so it is not that far of a reach to vary what age to start.

There is only one circumstance in which I would actually recommend avoiding fluoridated water for my own children: if they are exclusively formula fed under age one. Under age one, a child does not weigh as much, so it would not take as much fluoride to cause fluorosis. I would use nonfluoridated water if your child is exclusively formula fed, to help reduce the risk of fluorosis until age one. Bottled water is not guaranteed to be fluoride free, so you may have to order it from a water company or at a specialty baby store. I personally would switch back to fluoridated water after age twelve or eighteen months. We do not have any hard evidence on this either way.

ACID REFLUX

Acid reflux that goes away before age one is generally not a problem for teeth. Uncontrolled acid reflux after age one can be a significant problem for teeth. The longer it lasts, the worse it is. Acid reflux cuts out the "middleman"—carbohydrates. Instead of having bacteria produce acid to dissolve teeth, the acid from the stomach dissolves the teeth directly. Alternatively, a year or more of uncontrolled acid reflux may not cause the cavities per se, but it can sufficiently weaken the enamel so that cavities are close to inevitable. The best thing to do is to work with your doctor to try to control the acid reflux. If an acid reflux attack occurs, it is actually not a good idea to brush immediately afterward, because the enamel is in a weakened state after an acid episode. Drinking (or rinsing with) water after an acid attack is better. Alternatively, if your child is old enough to spit, swishing with a children's fluoride mouth rinse immediately afterward is beneficial because the acid causes the fluoride to incorporate into the teeth more easily. I wouldn't do more than two mouth rinses a day, however. If your child has had a history of acid reflux, starting a fluoride mouth rinse nightly is probably a good idea. I would also talk to your dentist about getting a prescription fluoride varnish applied every three months in the dental office for extra protection.

VITAMIN D

There is some good research that shows vitamin D can help prevent cavities, most likely by helping the teeth form with stronger enamel. Another way to say it is, a vitamin D deficiency could be a cause for 1–4 percent of the population getting what is called enamel hypoplasia, or really weak enamel. (We don't know for sure, but research does show a strong correlation.)

The only ways to get vitamin D are sunlight exposure or eating animal fats. Eggs, fish, many meats, and cod liver oil are all sources of vitamin D. Although cod liver oil works, it is pretty disgusting. Thankfully, milk is fortified with vitamin D. If your child does not drink dairy, or if you live in an area that is not very sunny, perhaps additional supplements could help.

I hesitate to give specific advice, because the research doesn't, so here is the best advice I can give.

1) Don't be afraid of all animal fats. Bacon and salmon both have vitamin D.
2) Get some sun, but not too much—not enough to get burned.
3) If your child lacks animal fats in the diet, or sunlight, consider vitamin D supplements.
4) You are probably good if you check your child's vitamin D levels with your doctor and aim for the recommended amount.

This could potentially include development of the teeth in utero, so I suppose pregnant women should go on vacation somewhere sunny. More practically, just be aware that maintaining adequate vitamin D levels may be important for normal tooth formation, so check with you medical doctor to see that your children are at the appropriate levels. They may recommend some infant drops if you live near me, in Seattle.

PREGNANCY

What should you do for your child's prenatal dental health? There is a lot that we don't know because it is inherently difficult to study cause and effect with prenatal development, but let's review a few of the basics.

See your dentist for regularly scheduled cleanings, and maintain good routine dental health. Periodontal disease in mothers has been linked with premature births. If you are actively following the prevention principles outlined in this book, my guess is that you won't have periodontal disease. Drinking more water helps everyone.

Talk to your dentist about what is elective and what is needed. Elective procedures can wait, but it is considered better to treat urgent dental needs while pregnant. Local anesthetic, x-rays, and other dental procedures have shown no apparent harm for pregnant women, but it is better to wait if treatment is considered elective. Talk with your dentist about what needs to be treated now and what can wait. Having an infection or bacteria enter the blood stream from a very large, untreated cavity could cause complications. After the first trimester is considered the best time to do any needed treatment.

As is true in general, make sure to take the recommended prenatal vitamins. Ask your doctor about vitamin D levels. As mentioned in the last chapter, try to get some sun while pregnant, as sunlight is an excellent source of vitamin D. Or eat more animal fat. Talk with your doctor about the current fish recommendations. Fish is an excellent source of vitamin D and omega-3 fatty acids, but you also want to limit mercury content at the same time.

If you do have cavities after your pregnancy, please feel no guilt whatsoever. This is a real occurrence, and you couldn't do anything about it. Morning sickness adds extra acid to the teeth. Trying to avoid morning sickness adds extra carbohydrates to the teeth. Changes in hormones and saliva cause issues with the teeth. As my wife says sarcastically, "every bad symptom is apparently normal if you are pregnant." You were creating life. Forgive yourself.

XYLITOL: WHY IT IS GOOD FOR TEETH

The three principles plus a tooth-friendly diet are the real keys to cavity prevention, but if you want to add a little extra prevention with gum or candy, xylitol is for you. Xylitol is a naturally occurring sugar alcohol derived originally from a Finnish tree sap. Bacteria that cause cavities cannot convert xylitol easily into lactic acid, similar to other sugar alcohols (such as mannitol or sorbitol). Xylitol tends to slow down bacteria better than other sugar alcohols.

The theory is that xylitol lowers the amount of bad bacteria, allowing more of the "good" bacteria to stay. One of the most fascinating studies was with Finnish mothers who chewed xylitol gum every day when their infants were between newborn and two years old. Having the mothers chew enough xylitol gum each day delayed the onset of cavities in their children by an average of three years. Researchers think that the xylitol-gum-chewing mothers had less of the bad mouth bacteria and therefore more of the good bacteria, which they passed on to their infants. Even with this information, I did not pressure my wife to chew xylitol gum. To replicate the study, she would have had to chew almost a pack of gum a day, which I think is not realistic.

However, I do chew a little every day because I will admit I don't brush my teeth after breakfast or lunch. Instead, I just chew a piece of xylitol gum for about ten seconds and then spit it out. If you chew gum already, I recommend switching to a 100 percent xylitol variety. There are also companies coming out with a wide assortment of xylitol candies, which can actually help prevent cavities instead of causing them!

THE SOCIAL CYCLE OF CAVITIES

Cavity formation and prevention has a definable social cycle that looks something like this:

- Dentist talks about prevention.
- Parent doesn't take the information too seriously because the child's teeth are baby teeth.
- Child gets cavities at age five or earlier.
- Parents feel guilty.
- Dentist doesn't want to make parents feel worse, so he says that some kids are high risk for cavities (or the dentist is still in the old drill-and-fill paradigm). Secretly they think flossing could have helped, when diet was more important.
- Parents do not learn from generations before them when it comes to cavities.

Here is how to break the cycle:

- Dentist talks about prevention in a way that makes sense and is easy to understand (based on diet first).
- Parents understand the importance of baby teeth.
- Parents follow the three principles and realize that diet is the key.
- Five-year-old is cavity-free, but are aware it was the snack foods.

- Parents feel empowered.
- Dentist feels happy preventing cavities with words (instead of drilling them away).
- Dentist does more one-year exams because it is even more educational and helpful for parents.
- Parents discuss importance of baby teeth with other parents.
- Every dentist (and every MD) knows the easy way to prevent cavities is by changing snack habits.
- Kids experience fewer needles and less trauma and pain.
- Younger siblings have a chance for zero cavities too.
- Then next generation of children has a chance for fewer cavities.

CLOSING THOUGHTS

The easiest way to prevent cavities is to start with the right habits as teeth emerge. This takes a paradigm shift because of common myths regarding children's teeth. But now that you understand that cavity formation comes down to diet, the stickiness of starches, and frequency of eating, you can make a difference. Discuss helpful information with your family and friends. Tell your dentist and pediatrician about it. Get passionate about good oral health because it contributes to good overall health.

Cavity prevention does not have to be complicated, but it does take different thinking. When your youngest child makes it to age five with zero cavities, e-mail me the good news that you were able to keep your whole family cavity-free so I, too, can share the reasons for your success with other parents. And give this manual for pediatric cavity prevention as a baby-shower gift so new parents can be successful, too.

REMEMBER, CAVITY PREVENTION STARTS AT THE GROCERY STORE.

Bibliography

Instead of the traditional reference section, I have decided to give a narrative of my references for the few of you who are interested. Most parents, please feel free to skip this section as you normally would. I write it for dentists in mind, so if you give this book to your dentist, he or she can check this section to see my reasoning for certain opinions. Of course, it is here for anyone to peruse. Any questions, please feel free to contact me. Even if you disagree with my reasoning, I appreciate feedback. My contact info is on TheDentistDad.com. Visit TheDentistDad.com/references for updated data.

Let's start out with some of the background data. It is confusing because different studies can cite different trends. I thought using the AAPD's most recent reference was appropriate. "The statistics are alarming. The rate of tooth decay in primary (baby) teeth of children aged 2 to 5 years increased nearly 17 percent from 1988–1994 to 1999–2004."

The American Academy of Pediatric Dentistry. "The State of Little Teeth." Aapd.org. AAPD, January 28, 2014. October 22, 2015. http://www.aapd.org/aapd%E2%80%99s_state_of_little_teeth_report_an_examination_of_the_epidemic_of_tooth_decay_among_our_youngest_children/.

Weston Price was one of the original dentists promoting diet as the cure for tooth decay. It is obvious that he was right. The problem with mainstream acceptance is three-fold. 1) Adoption of the low-fat diet as healthy. 2) It is highly impractical. 3) There was no valid hypothesis of why it worked, and the invalid explanations made no sense for modern scientists because they did not include bacteria in the equation. Weston Price found the cause, but did not account for the bacterial component so it could not be accepted by the mainstream. By combining the bacterial component with the anthropological studies, it finally makes sense. Eat more whole foods. Eat less processed carbohydrates. Eat more natural fats. Avoid sugars. My book aims to offer a practical alternative that is easy to do for busy moms.

Price, Weston A. *Nutrition and Physical Degeneration*. Lemon Grove, CA: Price-Pottenger Nutrition Foundation, 2008.

The following studies show how sugar-free gum after meals may help prevent cavities. This would make sense because anything that promotes saliva flow (which is stimulated by chewing) would help rinse away acids and increase remineralization. This is another good argument for chewing crunchy, raw vegetables: it promotes saliva flow.

Beiswanger, Bradley B., A. Elias Boneta, Melissa S. Mau, Barry P. Katz, Howard M. Proskin, and George K. Stookey. "The Effect Of Chewing Sugar-Free Gum After Meals On Clinical Caries Incidence." *The Journal of the American Dental Association* 129, no. 11 (1998): 1623–626.

Glass, R. L. "A Two-Year Clinical Trial of Sorbitol Chewing Gum." *Caries Res Caries Research* 17, no. 4 (1983): 365–68.

The below articles are very good references regarding biofilm. I was also reminded that bacteria need carbohydrates to be in aqueous form. This is why juice and dry flour mixed with saliva is worse than…quinoa.

Bowden, G. H. W., and Y. H. Li. "Nutritional Influences on Biofilm Development." *Advances in Dental Research* 11, no. 1 (1997): 81–99.

The following makes reference to complex carbohydrates being less cariogenic and refers to high concentrations of sucrose favoring *S. mutans*. It also discusses carbohydrates needing to be aqueous (diffusible) in oral plaque. Dentin has a critical pH value of 6.2 to 6.7.

Hara, Anderson T., and Domenick T. Zero. "The Caries Environment: Saliva, Pellicle, Diet, and Hard Tissue Ultrastructure." *Dental Clinics of North America* 54, no. 3 (2010): 455–67.

The following articles convinced me that we need to look at diet's affect on the virulence of bacteria and not simply look at bacteria without the influence of diet. Taking a sampling of bacteria is just a snapshot. The more frequent carbohydrate pulses, the more virulent the bacteria. If all glucose was taken away, *S. mutans* basically disappeared. Perhaps we should consider a strict low-carbohydrate diet for few days to reset patient's oral microflora, based on this in vitro study?

Bradshaw, D. H., A. S. McKee, and P. D. Marsh. "Effects of Carbohydrate Pulses and PH on Population Shifts within Oral Microbial Communities in Vitro." *Journal of Dental Research* 68, no. 9 (1989): 1298–302.

Fredrickson, A., and G. Stephanopoulos. "Microbial Competition." *Science* 213, no. 4511 (1981): 972–79.

The following article discusses the inverse correlation between calculus and caries rate. This makes sense because calculus comes from the minerals in the saliva, and saliva helps to rinse away acid and remineralize the tooth.

Duckworth, R. M., and E. Huntington. "On the Relationship between Calculus and Caries." *Monographs in Oral Science The Teeth and Their Environment* (2005): 1–28.

General good caries process references:

Fontana, Margherita, Douglas A. Young, Mark S. Wolff, Nigel B. Pitts, and Chris Longbottom. "Defining Dental Caries for 2010 and Beyond." *Dental Clinics of North America* 54, no. 3 (2010): 423–40.

González-Cabezas, Carlos. "The Chemistry Of Caries: Remineralization and Demineralization Events with Direct Clinical Relevance." *Dental Clinics of North America* 54, no. 3 (2010): 469–78.

Marsh, Philip D. "Microbiology of Dental Plaque Biofilms and Their Role in Oral Health and Caries." *Dental Clinics of North America* 54, no. 3 (2010): 441–54.

To be honest, I wasn't sure why the following article didn't make headline news. It wasn't even in the print edition of the AAPD journal. It was an e-article. The in-vitro studies are clear: low carbohydrate concentrations don't elicit the same acid response as high concentrations of carbohydrates. Increasing the fat concentration (as whole milk does) directly lowers the concentration of carbohydrates. Even skim milk was enough to lower acid, similar to sucrose! Whole milk did not. This article came out in the middle of my book writing and reinforced that I was on the right track in thinking that we shouldn't vilify fat the way we used to. Thankfully, the new dietary guidelines by the US in 2016 aren't as antifat as they used to be, so dentists should be less afraid to say, "Eat fat, not sugar or flour." Even though I specifically remember telling my mother to switch to skim milk while I was a teenager, I am now reversing gears, and am going to keep whole milk in the house for my children indefinitely, based on the higher sugar concentration of skim milk. That is not just for cavity prevention's sake, either.

Giacaman R. A., and C. Muñoz-Sandoval. "Cariogenicity of Different Commercially Available Bovine Milk Types in a Biofilm Caries Model." *Pediatric Dentistry* 36, no. 1 (2014): 1E–6E.

My favorite book on emotion coaching, which I referenced in the chapter on emotion coaching. The psychology aspect of teaching prevention is more important than the facts themselves, in my opinion. (Dr. Gottman does not endorse anything in my book. All opinions are based on my own interpretation of his book and listening to his lectures.)

Gottman, John Mordechai., and Joan DeClaire. *The Heart of Parenting: How to Raise an Emotionally Intelligent Child*. New York: Simon & Schuster, 1997.

Another good book for parents, from which I mention a concept on consistency (although that may have been from a lecture I attended):

Medina, John. Brain Rules for Baby: *How to Raise a Smart and Happy Child from Zero to Five*. Seattle: Pear, 2010.

The next article documents the only RCT study on humans that I am aware of, performed in the 1950s in Vipeholm. It's obviously not repeatable, but it is the best RCT we have, unfortunately. Frequency of sugar and stickiness were shown to be the most important variables with caries formation in our one RCT. All of the in-vitro science since then still supports those two variables, which is why I think we should put the most effort into teaching parents how to keep snack times organized. Obviously I am preaching to the choir, but my point is that if I had to choose one thing to focus on above all else, I would choose to teach parents to keep snack times organized first, then focus on the stickiness of starches, and then discuss all of the other variables after that. (Oral hygiene, fluoride, caries risk, genetics, and so on.) We tend to focus on brushing and fluoride first (which are important; don't get me wrong), but the science tells us frequency and stickiness (diet) are the *most* important.

Gustafsson, Bengt E., Carl-Erik Quensel, Lisa Swenander Lanke, Claes Lundqvist, Hans Grahnén, Bo Erik Bonow, and Bo Krasse. "The Effect of Different Levels of Carbohydrate Intake on Caries Activity in 436 Individuals Observed for Five Years." *Acta Odontol Scand Acta Odontologica Scandinavica* 11, no. 3–4 (1953): 232–364.

The following is a good study showing how breastfeeding correlates with a lower caries rate in a long-term study.

Hong, Liang, Steven M. Levy, DDS, MPH, John J. Warren, DDS, MS, and Barbara Broffitt, MS. "Infant Breast-feeding and Childhood Caries: A Nine-Year Study." *Pediatric Dentistry* 36, no. 4 (2014): 342–47.

In support of not using fluoridated water for bottle fed babies under age 1:

Walton, James L., and Louise B. Messer. "Dental Caries and Fluorosis in Breast-Fed and Bottle-Fed

Children." *Caries Res Caries Research* 15.2 (1981): 124-37.

Evidence that breast milk can contribute to caries formation if combined with other dietary carbohydrates, but otherwise does not:

Erickson, P. R., and E. Mazhari. "Investigation of the Role of Human Breast Milk in Caries Development." *Pediatr Dent.* 21.2 (1999): 86-90. <http://www.aapd.org/assets/1/25/Erickson-21-02.pdf>.

The following study is perhaps the most important and profound study of all. And it wasn't even done by dentists! This shows how much we know about the caries process. We know so much that the rate of demineralization can be explained by specific mathematical formulas that match very closely to clinical studies. This mathematical understanding again shows us that cavities are simply a calculus equation that is a function of (time), (carbohydrates), and (bacteria). However, (bacteria) only changes demineralization marginally compared to (time) and (carbohydrates). Once the carbohydrates are rinsed away, the acid is gone in twenty minutes. The buffering capacity of saliva has surprisingly little to do with things when we look at the math.

I love math because it is not emotional and is so difficult to argue with. This math model is another reason to prioritize our focus on organized eating and the stickiness of starches before all of the other good variables. If you are dentist and need to read one article on the caries process, this is what I would recommend to realize that it all comes down to math (and time):

Ilie, Olga, Mark C. M. Van Loosdrecht, and Cristian Picioreanu. "Mathematical Modelling of Tooth Demineralisation and PH Profiles in Dental Plaque." *Journal of Theoretical Biology* 309 (2012): 159–75.

Here's the definition of insidious—because crackers and dried flour are so sneaky.

Merriam-Webster. s.v. "Insidious." Accessed November 1, 2015. http://www.merriam-webster.com/.

The following study shows that most people can't guess what sticks to their teeth very well. The conclusion is that we should tell them (and it supports my reasoning for why handing out a stickiness-related snack guide is so important).

Kashket, S., J. Van Houte, L. R. Lopez, and S. Stocks. "Lack of Correlation Between Food Retention on the Human Dentition and Consumer Perception of Food Stickiness." *Journal of Dental Research* 70, no. 10 (1991): 1314–319.

This article discusses starches. When it comes down to it, starches cause cavities slower than sucrose; however, if they are very sticky, starches may be just as cariogenic because of the time factor. So juice all day can cause eight cavities in six months, but so can crackers all day.

Lingstrom, P., J. Van Houte, and S. Kashket. "Food Starches and Dental Caries." *Critical Reviews in Oral Biology & Medicine* 11, no. 3 (2000): 366–80.

Some good reviews of fluoride. The evidence is clear that fluoride can reduce cavities. However, I believe we should be focusing on the cause (diet) more than the medication. I still use fluoride for my children because we eat processed foods and lots of fruit, my daughter has weak enamel, and poor teeth genetics based on her parents:

Margolis, H. C., E. C. Moreno, and B. J. Murphy. "Effect of Low Levels of Fluoride in Solution on Enamel Demineralization in Vitro." *Journal of Dental Research* 65, no. 1 (1986): 23–29.

Bansal, Ankita, Navinanand Ingle, Navpreet Kaur, and Ekta Ingle. "Recent Advancements in Fluoride: A Systematic Review." *J Int Soc Prevent Communit*

Dent Journal of International Society of Preventive and Community Dentistry 5.5 (2015): 341. Web.

Classic study regarding the caries process:

Michalek, Suzanne M., Jerry R. McGhee, and Juan M. Navia. "Virulence of Streptococcus Mutans: A Sensitive Method for Evaluating Cariogenicity in Young Gnotobiotic Rats." *Infection and Immunicty* 12, no. 1 (1975): 69–75.

A great chapter on diet and dental caries epidemiology:

National Research Council (US) Committee on Diet and Health. "Dental Caries. Diet and *Health: Implications for Reducing Chronic Disease Risk.* US National Library of Medicine, 1989. December 27, 2015. http://www.ncbi.nlm.nih.gov/books/NBK218734/.

The tragic story of Deamonte Driver:

Otto, Mary. "For Want of a Dentist." *The Washington Post*, February 27, 2007.http://www.washington-post.com/wp-dyn/content/article/2007/02/27/AR2007022702116.html.

A correlation between early dental visits and reduction in cavities:

Savage, M. F. "Early Preventive Dental Visits: Effects on Subsequent Utilization and Costs." *Pediatrics* 114, no. 4 (2004): n.p.

Here is the meta-analysis that shows no link between flossing and caries reduction. It actually shows more caries instead of less:

Dental Flossing and Interproximal Caries: a Systematic Review P.P. Hujoel, J. Cunha-Cruz, D.W. Banting and W.J. Loesche J DENT RES 2006; 85; 298

Here is the meta-analysis on vitamin D reducing caries rates.

Hujoel, Philippe P. "Vitamin D and Dental Caries in Controlled Clinical Trials: Systematic Review and Meta-analysis." *Nutr Rev Nutrition Reviews* 71.2 (2012): 88-97. Web.

Here is an article by Dr. Hujoel discussing how cavities and overall health can be linked by diet.

Hujoel, P. "Dietary Carbohydrates and Dental-Systemic Diseases." *Journal of Dental Research* 88.6 (2009): 490-502.

Made in the USA
Charleston, SC
09 December 2016